MW00962061

Keto Diet for Beginners
&
Keto Meal Prep

2 IN 1

Easy and Complete Weight Loss Guide With a Stunning Collection of Quick and Delicious, Low Carb Ketogenic Recipes to Prep, Grab, and Go!

Serena Baker

Additionally, the information in the following pages is intended only for informational purposes and should thus be thought of as universal. As befitting its nature, it is presented without assurance regarding its prolonged validity or interim quality. Trademarks that are mentioned are done without written consent and can in no way be considered an endorsement from the trademark holder.

Keto Diet for Beginners:

Easy and Complete Weight Loss Guide to a High-Fat/Low-Carb Lifestyle.

Reset your Health With these Ketogenic-Fasting Ideas, and add more Clarity and Confidence in your Life!

By Serena Baker

Introduction

Congratulations on beginning your journey to weight loss, health, and feeling great! At first glance, the ketogenic diet seems overwhelming and complicated. People think it's not something they can stick with, or share with friends and family. But the reality is it's a lot easier than you think! In this book, we are going to hold your hand and take you step-by-step through the ketogenic diet. First, we'll give an overview of what the diet is and how it works. Then we'll review the benefits of the diet. After we've got all the basics covered, we'll tell you exactly what you need to know in order to get started! We'll give you an eating plan and recipes. Not sure what to eat for breakfast? We've got you covered! And lunch and dinner too.

The ketogenic diet is quite easy to follow. It seems like a diet you won't be able to fit in with your friends when they want to go out to eat, but nothing could be further from the truth. If you're just a little bit careful, following the keto diet (as it's known for short) is very easy. So, let's get started!

Chapter 1: An Overview of the Ketogenic Diet

If you're like me, then for years you've been completely brainwashed. Nutrition experts, doctors, and dieticians all said the same thing – Eat a low-fat diet! They told us that fat put the weight on, raised our cholesterol, and caused heart attacks.

A funny thing happened – none of that turned out to be true. After years of telling everyone that they needed to eat a high-carbohydrate and low-fat diet, doctors began noticing something strange. People were putting on weight! And nobody was getting any healthier. At first, they thought it was because people couldn't stick to diets. And there was some truth to that. After all, dieting using the old scheme required calorie counting and deprivation. Most of us found that got old fast. When the hunger pains came, we dove in.

Finally, it began dawning on people maybe something wasn't right. Years ago, Dr. Atkins had been urging people to eat low carb. Some were doing it, but the vast majority of doctors thought it was nutty. But as the experts started learning about diabetes and the way the body worked, they began to realize that Atkins was onto something and that the low-fat diet idea was wrong.

What Is the Ketogenic Diet?

The ketogenic diet is a high-fat, moderate-protein, and low-carb diet. There's nothing very complicated about it. It's a little bit different, than the standard low-carb dieting you've heard about, because generally people on low-carb haven't worried about their protein intake. With keto, you eat proteins in adequate amounts but keep them in check. We'll see why that's the case in a bit.

But what about all that fat? Is it going to clog my arteries?

The answer for most people is a resounding *no*. The ketogenic diet is based on a diet of healthy fats. You probably already know the standard litany – omega-3's in fish, and olive oil are right for you, but animal fat, not so much.

Well, guess what. That turned out not to be true either.

Yes, it is true that olive oil is right for you. And so are fish. But what about animal fat? Well about five years ago or so researchers got a big shock. When the saturated fat found in animal meats was studied in detail – they found out it didn't raise heart attack risk at all.

So, it's safe to eat a fatty cut of steak. In fact, we encourage it. Basically, you can think of saturated fat as the neutral fat, and olive oil and fish oil are the best fats. It turned out that saturated fat only causes health problems when it's consumed in a diet heavy on carbs. When you're eating low carb, it's just fine. So, go ahead and have some steak and lamb, and add some butter if you want to.

The History of the Ketogenic Diet

The ketogenic diet traces its roots to the treatment of epilepsy. Surprisingly this goes all the way back to 500 BC, when ancient Greeks observed that fasting or eating a ketogenic diet helped reduce epileptic seizures. In modern times, the ketogenic diet was reintroduced in the practice of medicine to treat children with epilepsy. In 1921, a scientist named Rollin Woodyatt discovered that the liver made ketone bodies during starvation or when the patient was following a high fat, low carbohydrate diet.

Research into the keto diet stalled until the 1960s, when scientists discovered that a certain class of fats called *medium chain triglycerides* or MCTs were readily transported to the liver and made into ketone bodies, faster than normal fats (coconut oil is an example). It was also found that the body could go into a state of ketosis eating more protein when large amounts of MCTs were consumed.

In the early 1970s, a cardiologist named Robert Atkins proposed his own version of a ketogenic diet called the Atkins diet, which has been immensely popular. The Atkins diet has more relaxed standards that keto, allowing adherents to follow very strict carbohydrate consumption for the first two weeks during an "induction phase." After this, the number of carbohydrates consumed can be slightly increased.

From there, research on ketogenic diets stalled again. However, in the past fifteen years, there has been an explosion of interest in the diet.

How Keto Is Different from Other Diets

It's obvious how keto is different from many diets. The standard American way of dieting is to eat a high carb diet while restricting fats. Extensive calorie counting is required. It can be said that the keto diet is the opposite of the standard method of dieting.

Another popular diet is the Mediterranean diet. This diet, which is based on the eating habits of people who live along the

Mediterranean Sea, is based on a varied diet including fish, whole grains, nuts, fruits, vegetables, cheese, and occasional meat. Legumes also play a central role in the menu. Many health benefits are ascribed to the keto diet but it still involves the consumption of large amounts of carbohydrates, so may not work well for those who are attracted to the keto diet.

There are many other low carbohydrate diets on the market. We've already mentioned the Atkins diet, which has been very popular and kept the keto-eating pattern alive in the public mind. The keto diet is stricter than Atkins. As we mentioned above, Atkins allows dieters to limit carbohydrate consumption to 20 grams a day for the first two weeks. After that, they can gradually add more carbs to their diet up to a point. The keto diet is different in that you cannot start adding carbs to the diet. Some people may find they do better eating carbs at a higher level, but generally speaking, a keto diet is a lifestyle change rather than a temporary "diet." Another difference between keto and Atkins is that Atkins doesn't place formal limits on protein intake; its focus is only on limiting the number of carbs consumed daily.

The *Paleo diet* claims to be based on the eating patterns of pre-historical peoples. Whether this is true or not we'll leave to the anthropologists to figure out, but paleo (and an offshoot known as "primal") is a style of low carb eating that is someone more relaxed than Atkins and ketogenic dieting. Paleo allows the consumption of specific high fiber but high carb foods like sweet potatoes that are not allowed on keto. Many paleo adherents also eat nuts and berries, which adds more carbs to the diet than what would probably be considered appropriate on keto. However, the paleo diet is quite a change from the standard American diet.

The South Beach Diet is another low carb diet, which is really an offshoot of the Atkins diet. The difference is Atkins, at least as initially proposed, allow people to eat any amount of fat they like. South Beach attempted to combine the popular notion of eating lean proteins with a low carb diet. It works for some people, but if you are trying to get by on low carbs with low-fat meals, you'll probably find yourself hungry, lacking mental clarity, and feeling unsatisfied.

On the other end of the spectrum, we have the *Ornish* diet, vegetarians, and veganism. The Ornish diet takes standard dieting advice to the extreme, favoring low glycemic carbohydrates in large amounts and severely restricting fat intake, to less than 10% of calories.

At first sight, the vegetarian and vegan diets might seem the opposite of keto, but in fact, you can be a vegetarian and still enjoy a keto diet. The hard part is getting vegetarian protein sources that are also low in carbs. However, many oils can be safely consumed like olive oil, and you can eat all the avocados you like.

The Science Behind the Ketogenic Diet

Researchers are starting to build a large amount of evidence that supports the ketogenic diet. In 2004, an article titled "Long-term effects of a ketogenic diet in obese patients" was published in Experimental Clinical Cardiology. The researchers found that a 24-week diet that limited daily carbohydrate intake to 30 grams and total protein intake to one gram per pound of body weight resulted in significant weight loss among participants. The patients in the study also saw improved lipid profiles, with increasing HDL or "good" cholesterol and decreased levels of LDL or "bad" cholesterol, triglycerides, and blood sugar. Later researchers have confirmed that a ketogenic diet leads to significant weight loss when studied in a controlled setting, while also providing other benefits such as better blood sugar control.

What Are the Health Benefits of a Ketogenic Diet?

The first benefit of the ketogenic diet is weight loss. When you start keto, if you actually stick to it, you're going to lose weight rapidly. With no carbs to burn for fuel, your body turns to burn fat – including *your fat*. And for reasons that we'll explain in a minute, you'll also get rid of unwanted water weight.

If it stopped there, the keto diet would be a wondrous thing. But we're just getting started – the keto diet has many benefits. First, let's talk about diabetes.

In many western societies, especially in the United States, diabetes is at epidemic levels. The culprit is our diets – and it's not what they thought it was. You're probably guessing by now it wasn't fat, *it was the carbs*. For people with the genetic tendency, eating a carbohydrate diet made them gain weight and set them up for diabetes.

That's where the keto diet comes in. Health benefit number two is it lowers your blood sugar and often does so dramatically. If you're pre-diabetic or diabetic (type 2), you may be shocked with the results you get doing keto. Your fasting blood sugars are going to drop, and you'll see lower A1c scores as well. For some, they've even dropped into the normal range. If you're pre-diabetic and not on any meds, you can probably manage this yourself. But if you already have diabetes and take medications, be sure to discuss your keto eating plan with your doctor. Your dropping blood sugar might mean you need to dial back your medications or insulin.

Speaking of insulin, many people who don't have diabetes develop insulin resistance as they become middle-aged. They get a little pudgy around the middle, and when they eat a high carb meal, their cells just don't work right. The pancreas releases the insulin it's supposed to, but the cells don't quite respond. They've become *insulin resistant*. More insulin needs to be released to get them to take up the sugar. The good news is a keto diet will lower insulin resistance.

Another benefit of the keto diet is that directly lowers your risk of heart disease. Crazy right? Eating all that fat and you have a *lower* risk of heart attack? That almost seems like a magic trick. Here's how it does it – triglycerides. While doctors were fretting about total cholesterol, they didn't notice all those people with normal cholesterol levels having heart attacks. What was going on?

First a brief overview of blood fats. Cholesterol is transported through the body using *lipoproteins*. This is a molecule made up of fat ("lipo") and protein. There are two significant types of cholesterol you need to be concerned about, which are classified by their density, or how crowded they are packed. One is low density or LDL, and the other is high density, or HDL. Traditionally we've been told that a high cholesterol number is not good for you, but after decades of research, scientists have discovered that this designation is simplistic. Half of all first time heart attack victims have supposedly healthy levels of total cholesterol.

LDL was believed to be the culprit behind heart disease, and this is true to a degree, but the picture is not as simple as once believed. However, the legacy belief that its bad for you has led to the designation that LDL is "bad cholesterol." For years, doctors have believed that just by controlling LDL levels, they could reduce heart disease risk.

It turns out that there are many risk factors for heart disease, and one little-noticed lipid problem is the amount of triglycerides in your blood, which is a type of blood fat. More specifically, your heart disease risk is accurately determined from the ratio of triglycerides to HDL.

Triglycerides are blood fats the liver makes after a meal, usually one heavy in carbohydrates. A large amount of triglycerides are also produced by the liver when an excess amount of alcohol is consumed.

HDL is also known as "good cholesterol." Its job is to clean out excess LDL or "bad cholesterol" from the arteries. Next time you get blood labs done get your numbers and do a little calculation if they don't do it for you. Divide your triglyceride number by the HDL number. If it's less than three, you're OK. Ideally, it should be close to one. However, if it's greater than three, you have a high risk of having a future heart attack.

Luckily the keto diet steps up to the plate again. When you follow a keto lifestyle, you'll see your triglycerides drop. Many people see utterly dramatic results. For many, HDL also increases. So, keto will lower your triglyceride to HDL ratio and dramatically decrease your risk of heart attack.

If that were all keto did, we'd be happy, but it turns out higher insulin levels in the body can also raise blood pressure. That's a terrible thing – high blood pressure can lead to many serious health problems. It raises your risk of stroke and heart attack, as well as putting you at risk for kidney damage and other issues.

One reason this happens is raised insulin levels can cause water and salt retention. And that leads to high blood pressure. The good news is that by lowering your insulin levels, keto leads to lower blood pressure values in many people.

Insulin also acts as a fat storing hormone. When you're eating a high-carbohydrate diet, all that insulin flowing around is going to tell your body to store the sugar in fat cells. This is how high carbohydrate diets can make people gain weight even if they are eating low fat and "watching the calories." If we keep blood sugars stable and level, there is less insulin released, and as a result, the body will store less fat. The healthy way to achieve this result is to eat a keto diet.

Keto has also been shown to improve mental health. This isn't surprising, for nearly a century it's been used to treat epilepsy in children. So, doctors have known for some time that keto diets had an impact on the nervous system. Now many people are reporting more stable moods, less depression, and higher concentration on keto.

Keto diets can also help with sleep and digestion problems. The reason for this is that the blood sugar spikes that you get while on a typical western diet high in carbs won't be happening anymore. With keto, your blood sugar will be steady as she goes at all times. This also helps with mood and anxiety as well.

Ketosis: A Detailed Overview

Usually our bodies use sugar for energy. Blood sugar rises after a meal is digested, and then insulin is released. Insulin tells your cells to take up the sugar. You can think of insulin as a signal or as a key that opens a door. Once the cells take up the sugar, they can process it to obtain energy and your blood sugar drops back down to background levels.

As we age and gain weight, our cells become insulin resistant. This means that they are less responsive to the hormone insulin, so won't take up as much sugar. The blood sugar in the body rises, and this creates a large number of health problems. Blood sugar can damage your blood vessels and left unchecked high blood sugar levels can cause kidney failure, blindness, heart disease, stroke, and other problems like erectile dysfunction.
Early on there probably aren't any symptoms at all, and you'll only notice that you're putting on weight every year. Maybe you feel a little more fatigued, and if it continues to get worse, you might find yourself drinking more water.

As insulin resistance develops, the body tries to compensate by releasing more insulin. This sets up a deadly cycle. Over time more and more insulin needs to be produced to keep up.

To avoid the deadly cycle, we can rely on metabolizing fats instead. It turns out that sugar isn't the only fuel the body can run on. When you're either fasting or your body is low on sugar, the body can produce fuel from another source by burning fats for energy. This process is called *ketosis*.

Ketosis works by using three molecules that scientists call acetoacetate, beta-hydroxybutyrate, and acetone. If that gave you a momentary headache don't worry about it! To understand ketosis you don't have to know the actual names of the molecules. All you need to know is that the body can utilize these three ketones for energy in place of sugar. When ketones are found in the blood, the body is said to be in a state of *ketosis*.

Under certain circumstances, the liver will convert fat into ketones. When the liver releases ketones, they enter the bloodstream and are distributed throughout the body where they can be used by the cells as fuel.

Something important to know is that too much protein will inhibit this process. This is because the body can make glucose (blood sugar) from protein, and it will do so when actual sugar is in short supply. Overeating protein is often a reason that people "hit a wall" when attempting low-carb diets such as Paleo or Atkins. They eat too much protein and end up keeping their blood sugar levels high, and fail to enter ketosis. The result is they are unable to lose weight.

So, keep this rule in mind: eat adequate protein but only eat protein in moderation.

The question before us is how do we put the body into a state of ketosis. The way to do it is to deplete your sugar levels. The uncomfortable way to do it is to go through a period of fasting. When you're not eating anything, you're not eating carbs either, and you'll go into ketosis. Some people do incorporate fasting into their keto program, and that may be an option for you. However it's not necessary, and you can still achieve the same results without starving yourself.

How? By eating a diet with moderate amounts of proteins, very low carbs and high levels of fats – we naturally put the body in a state of ketosis.

While you don't have to do it, many people are interested in actually finding out if they are in ketosis. You can buy and handheld meter and find out. The meter will report the level of ketones in your blood. Ketones are measured in units of mmol/L. It is recommended that your ketone level is in the range of 1.5-3.0 mmol/L. This is the "optimal" range which will help you achieve your weight loss goals. If your ketone level is below this range, then you need to take a closer look at your diet. First, make sure you're not eating too much protein. If that isn't the culprit, then look at your total carbs and see if you can reduce them.

A ketone test kit can be purchased online for around $50-$70.

People doing keto for the first time may experience some unpleasant side effects when going into ketosis. The most common symptoms are feeling "under the weather." Some people call this the "keto flu," and it's characterized by lethargy, possible headaches, and irritability. Some people will also experience constipation, and others may experience heart palpitations.

The best way to avoid these problems is to do the following: make sure you're getting enough water and enough key minerals. You may need to drink more water than you're used to, at least at first. Other problems, in particular, heart palpitations, maybe caused by a failure to get adequate minerals. Two key minerals you should focus on are potassium and magnesium. You can take supplements, but the problem with potassium is that they only come in 99 mg pills and the daily requirement is in the thousands of mg. The best way to get potassium is from your diet. Meat does supply some potassium, and you can also get it from leafy green vegetables and broccoli. If you find out or feel your potassium level is low, consider adding spinach, arugula, or kale to your eating plans.

You can use magnesium supplementation. It is often available in 250 mg or 500 mg doses. You'll want to take a maximum of 500 mg per day. Magnesium helps a great deal with heart palpitations, maintaining proper blood pressure, and avoiding constipation.

But here's a tip. Eat avocados. This lush fruit is mostly fat, and it's mainly good monounsaturated fats. But for our purposes here the key fact about avocados is that they contain ample amounts of vitamins and minerals. Checking the nutrition facts, we find that one cup of sliced avocado supplies 24% of your vitamin c needs, 20% of vitamin B-6, 10% of magnesium, and 20% of daily recommended potassium. That cup of avocado only has 2 grams of net carbs as well – so it fits in with a keto diet.

That brings up an important aside, how do you calculate net carbs? It's very easy. Only note the total carbs and the dietary fiber. Subtract dietary fiber from total carbohydrates. That's the net carbs for any food.

Now let's turn to a thorny issue – *ketoacidosis*. First, let's be clear that ketoacidosis is not something you have to worry about at all. But we have to bring it up because it sounds like ketosis and people often confuse the two processes. But they are not the same and are not caused by similar processes. Ketosis is a normal process used by the body. Ketoacidosis is a dysfunctional situation.

First off, ketoacidosis is only of concern for diabetics – and chiefly those with type 1 diabetes. If you don't have type 1 diabetes, you shouldn't be worrying about ketoacidosis.

Ketoacidosis is a malfunction that occurs when the level of ketone bodies in your system reaches 10-15 mmol/L. This can cause stomach pain, nausea, and vomiting. Higher levels can result in confusion and even coma or death.

However, when you're following a ketogenic diet, you're likely to max out at a ketone body level of 3 mmol/L, a level much lower than that seen with ketoacidosis. Reasonably healthy people can maintain levels of ketone bodies within safe levels very easily. This is because your pancreas will release insulin if ketone bodies get too high, and this will signal the liver to stop making them.

That's why type 1 diabetics have to worry about ketoacidosis. Their bodies can't produce insulin, so could not shut down a runaway ketone body problem. For most of us, this is not something we need to worry about.

However, there are two cases where ketoacidosis could be a concern even if you don't have type 1 diabetes. This is when you have type 2 diabetes and taking certain medications, or you're breastfeeding. If you're breastfeeding, you may want to discuss a keto diet with your doctor first. Complications with breastfeeding and keto are rare, however.

In the case of type 2 diabetes, those taking the medications Farxiga, Jardiance, or Invokana (or other SGLT-2 inhibitors) may be at risk of ketoacidosis if they go on a ketogenic diet. If you have type 2 diabetes and taking one of these drugs, please speak to your doctor first. It may be important to discontinue the medication before going on a diet.

In any case, if you're breastfeeding or a person with type 2 diabetes taking one of these medications and you suspect that you're showing the symptoms of ketoacidosis, eat some carbohydrates. This will help release insulin and stop the process. Then call 911. It's also good to have a ketosis meter on hand so you can check your blood level of ketones.

A surprising fact about ketones is that they're brain food. Many people (including some doctors) mistakenly believe that the brain must have blood sugar for energy. The truth is that is not the case. The brain is perfectly happy burning ketones for power, and there is some evidence that this is better for the brain. Ketone bodies may help the brain function better and stabilize moods.

To maximize weight loss, you'll want to optimize ketosis. This means that you should have ketone bodies in the range of 1.5-3.0 mmol/L. If you are in the range 0.5-1.5 mmol/L, you're said to be in "light ketosis." That's better than not being in ketosis at all, but you want it in that 1.5-3.0 mmol/L range. If you're not in the optimal range first, make sure your carb intake is as low as you want it to be. It's a good idea to keep a journal or record of your food consumption, so you know exactly how many carbs you're consuming. You'll also want to note the number of grams of protein per day, since overeating protein will result in the liver making glucose, raising your blood sugar levels. This will inhibit ketosis and inhibit weight loss.

Determining If Keto Is Right for You

You wouldn't be reading this book if you weren't interested in losing weight and improving your cardiovascular health. But is keto for everyone? It turns out it's not, but keto should work out for most people. The best way to determine if keto is right for you is to see if you are one of the people who *shouldn't* be on keto. If you're not in one of those groups, then keto is right for you after all. So, who are the people that shouldn't be on keto?

There are no hard and fast rules, but we can consider the following:

- High blood pressure. If you have high blood pressure keto may not work for you. However, it will probably work out fine for most people with high blood pressure, in fact, it will probably help them get off their medications by causing weight loss and also some loss of body fluids and the associated excess salt. But you should realize that keto can lower your high blood
- pressure, and if you're on medications that can cause some problems. You should discuss this with your doctor. If you start keto and your blood pressure drops, your doctor may have to adjust your medication dosage. But that's what we're hoping for anyway!

- Breastfeeding. In rare cases, breastfeeding moms can run into trouble while on keto. Discuss with your doctor first.

- People with type 2 diabetes. With type 2 diabetics, there are two areas of concern. Your blood sugar levels may drop eliminating the necessity of medications like metformin. If you're using insulin, dosages will need to be reduced or even eliminated since you're not consuming carbs. As noted above, if you're taking an SGLT-2 inhibitor like Farxiga, you may be at risk of ketoacidosis. In all cases speak with your doctor about these issues before doing a keto diet.

- People with type 1 diabetes.

If you're not in one of those groups, then you should be good to go with a keto diet. The only issue once we've cleared up possible health risks is making sure that you're disciplined enough. Are you unable to give up carbs, period? If so, then maybe the keto diet isn't for you. That doesn't mean you can't have an occasional lapse or even now and then cheat day, but those who want to keep eating everything probably shouldn't go on keto. Do you value potato chips and the occasional slice of bread or losing weight more? Ask yourself and then act appropriately.

Pros and Cons of the Keto Diet

Quite frankly the advantages of the keto diet are easy. We've already discussed many of them. Let's list them here:

- You'll lose weight and look better.
- Lose body fat.
- More energy.
- Mental clarity.
- Stable moods.
- Risk of heart disease will drop.
- Risk of stroke will drop.
- Risk of some cancers related to obesity will drop.
- You'll sleep better.
- You'll reduce acid reflux if you have it.
- You'll reduce acne if you have it.
- Blood sugar will be reduced.
- If you're pre-diabetic, you'll probably cure it.
- If your diabetic you'll probably cut your A1C, and some may be able to get off medication.
- Your blood lipids will improve.
- If you're suffering from non-alcoholic fatty liver disease, going on keto will cure it.
- You'll think less about food.

- A keto diet may reduce the risk of cancer.

That's a long list, and we've probably missed a few things. But we'd be lying if we said that keto was the perfect diet. There are some cons of the keto diet.

- Lethargy or headaches. Most likely due to "keto flu." Make sure you're drinking enough water. Also, check your mineral intake.

- Dry mouth. Results from not enough water. It's sometimes recommended to drink a cup of bullion each day, to help your body maintain proper salt levels (remember keto causes fluid loss, salt goes with it).

- Increased urination. When you first adapt to keto, you might urinate more than usual. This effect is usually temporary.

- Bad breath. This results from acetone in your breath and sometimes in your sweat. Usually temporary.

- Reduced exercise performance. If you're a pro-athlete, you may have issues with reduced performance from a lack of carbs.

So, what's the verdict? We vote yes on the keto diet. Most of the downsides are minor and temporary.

Issues That May Come Up with a High Fat Diet

Most issues that come up with a high fat diet like keto result from beginners' mistakes. Your body is used to balance it gets via minerals and fiber in foods like pasta and bread. When you suddenly stop eating these foods, without adequate replacements you may run into issues.

One of the most common issues that comes up on a high fat diet like keto is constipation. There are three main reasons for this that you can look into if this happens to you. The first is to make sure you're getting adequate water intake. The second issue you may face is not getting enough fiber. To increase fiber, look at adding some low carb vegetables to your meal plans. Spinach, kale, arugula, cauliflower, and broccoli are excellent choices. You may also consider avocado, which is packed with both fiber and essential minerals. But please be aware of the calories contained in avocado. Finally, check your magnesium.

Heart palpitations are a common problem for beginners in high-fat diets. Typically, these result from an easily corrected mineral imbalance. The usual culprit, in this case, is magnesium. You can either address it by adding magnesium-rich fruits and vegetables to your diet or by using supplements.

Irritability and brain fog are also common complaints when starting keto. Usually, these are temporary problems as your body adjusts. If they continue to make sure your water intake and minerals are where they need to be.

Muscle loss is an unexpected issue that may come up with some keto dieters. While it's important to consume protein in moderate quantities, some people end up eating too little protein. Make sure you get adequate amounts of protein, especially if you're someone who works out.

Tips and Tricks for Transitioning to a Keto Lifestyle

Now let's have a look at some tips that will help you adapt to a keto lifestyle successfully. The first thing to remember is that for most people, this style of eating is a significant change in their lives. So, the first thing you need to bring to the table is a firm commitment to losing weight and improving your health. If you're the kind of person who is going to be easily tempted by cheating, the keto lifestyle may not be for you. But if you've committed, let's forge ahead.

One tip is to get a friend to go on keto with you. It helps to have a support system, and while you can (and should) get online to talk to others also starting on a keto diet for support and to exchange ideas, it helps to have a personal friend involved. You may already have some friends trying out a keto diet or others who are thinking about it. Talk to them and find out. If you can do it together the added support will help you stay on a diet.

Next, make sure you familiarize yourself with the potential pitfalls that you might face while starting out a keto diet. One way to deal with this is to keep a journal. Drinking adequate water – alone – is one of the most important things that beginners can do to avoid problems. You should keep a journal that tracks how many glasses of water you're drinking daily. That way you can precisely plan how to proceed if you're showing symptoms like dry mouth or headaches that could indicate inadequate water intake.

You can use your journal or diary for other purposes too, such as tracking the amount of protein and carbohydrate consumed each day. By writing down everything, you eat it will be easy to pinpoint problem areas.

Our next tip is don't wait for problems to arise. Make sure you have important supplements in hand before you go full blown with a ketogenic diet. Magnesium may be a vital supplement you need to get a good brand of 250 mg or 500 mg magnesium supplements to have on hand in case you start showing symptoms of problems. In fact, that level of magnesium dosage is virtually harmless while providing many benefits, so it wouldn't hurt to simply add at least 250 mg to your diet right away. This can help keep you "regular" and avoid more concerning problems like heart palpitations.

Sleep is vital for all of us, and that's especially the case when making a major change in your life. And keto is a significant change for most people. Make sure you carve out time to get your beauty rest! And, make sure you have a comfortable mattress and don't take your smartphone to bet with you!

Get some exercise. Even if you don't feel like it because keto is making you feel low energy, moderate exercise can go a long way in helping your body overcome problems like irritability and keto flu quickly. You don't need to kill yourself either. Just add a 30-minute walk to your daily routine.

Monitor your progress. Weigh yourself frequently but not daily. Also, if you can afford to do so, buy a ketone monitor so you'll know if you're really in keto or not. There is no sense guessing when the technology to find out is readily available.

Running into a wall? How often do you hear people who are dieting that stop making progress? If you do keto right and follow it carefully, this shouldn't happen. But if it does – consider taking a day off. Just don't make it a habit. But a single day off where you eat all the carbs you want can help your body reset and over the long term, you'll lose more weight. Don't let it become a trap. However, the idea of a day off might turn into two days off, then three or more if you're not a disciplined personality type. Limit yourself to a maximum of two days off per month.

Chapter 2: Starting the Ketogenic Diet

Now you have an idea of what the keto diet is all about, what ketogenesis is and what the pitfalls are. It's time to get started!

How to Start a Keto Diet

The first step in starting a diet is to compile a food list. It's quite simple to get started. The first thing is to note your protein limit. It's good to keep a notebook, so you don't stray outside your boundaries and run into roadblocks.

The general rule of thumb is to keep protein consumption to 0.45-0.5 grams of protein per pound of body weight per day. So, if you weigh 160 pounds, the amount of protein you should eat per day is 80 grams. That's a fair amount of protein. On the inside of your notebook write down your starting weight and a few reminders, like the protein limit per day and a list of prohibited foods.

Now that you know how much protein you can eat per day, what sources of protein are allowed? Virtually everything!

- All animal protein is allowed. Just make sure you're observing your daily protein limit.

- All seafood is allowed. You'll want to seek out high-fat fish, like salmon, swordfish, tuna, mackerel, and sardines. You can eat lean seafood as well but watch that protein count and be sure to pair it with other high-fat food items like avocado.

- In the early stages at least, avoid nuts. Avoid fruits and berries at all cost.

- No bread, wheat, pasta, rice, or potatoes. That includes sweet potatoes.

- Eat leafy green vegetables, cauliflower, and broccoli. But remember they do contain some carbs so don't eat unlimited amounts.

- Avoid tomatoes, at least for the first couple of months.

- Try using coconut oil and coconut cream, good sources of MCT fats.

- Avocados are an excellent addition to a ketogenic diet. An avocado is a fruit but very low in carbs and high in fat. Also provides many essential vitamins and minerals.

Who Benefits the Most from a Ketogenic Diet?

Who benefits from the keto diet? Anyone who wants to lose weight! But certain people in particular, will really excel on the keto diet. The first group of people is those who simply end up starting a diet like Atkins and then hitting a wall. If you try a diet like that and you start losing weight but find yourself stagnant or even gaining weight back a couple of weeks later, then keto might be a better option for you. You will benefit from the keto diet because it keeps proteins in check better than Atkins, South Beach, and the paleo diet.

People will slow metabolisms (that don't have documented thyroid problems) will benefit from keto. It's possible your slow metabolism is a result of problems with digesting and processing carbohydrates.

Prediabetics are probably the number one group of people that benefit on the keto diet. If you haven't been diagnosed with diabetes yet but tend to have high fasting blood sugars and you're gaining weight around your midsection but don't have any other serious health problems, then the keto diet is definitely one you will benefit from. The keto diet will normalize your blood sugars, help you lose weight fast and correct other metabolic problems often associated with prediabetes.

Type 2 diabetics can also benefit from the keto diet. But go over the possible risks that we discussed in the previous chapter, and always be sure to consult the ketogenic diet with your doctor before starting it.

Finally, let's note that both men and women benefit from the keto diet. If you need to lose weight, it doesn't matter what your gender is.

Avoiding Common Beginner's Mistakes

To avoid common beginner mistakes, the first advice is to track your activities, at least for the first couple of weeks. Some tips are:

- Drink adequate amounts of water. Use your intuition to know if you're getting enough water or not. If you find yourself having dry mouth problems, drink more.

- Make sure you're not going over your protein limits. This is the most common mistake made with keto. Remember that if you eat more than 0.5 grams of protein per pound of your body weight per day, your liver will convert some protein into blood sugar ruining the diet. Be sure to track this accurately, as you lose weight you might need to cut back on protein some more.

- Plan ahead for eating out. Don't let yourself get into a situation where "cheating" becomes necessary by eating a sandwich or slice of pizza.

- Watch for hidden carbs. Another common mistake made by beginners is to eat some fatty meat, but pile on some sugary sauces with it. Unfortunately, many favorites like barbecue sauce or teriyaki sauce can be loaded with sugar. When eating at home be sure to include the counts of carbohydrates in any sauces you use toward your total daily limit. When eating out, you can run into trouble because you may not know how many carbs are in a given sauce or salad dressing.

- Hidden carbs you may not be thinking of. You might think of cream or half and half as fatty. And they are – but they also contain carbohydrates. The amount of carbohydrates is minimal, but you need to keep track of every gram. And if you decide to consume a large amount of cream, you're going to need to know how many carbs you're dragging along. Cream is better than half-and-half, which is the watered-down version that retains the carbohydrates with less fat.

- Don't overeat fat. This advice might strike you as odd since we've been singing the praises of following a high fat diet plan! But it's true, calories still matter and you can overdo it with the fat as well. But this isn't weight watchers. You don't have to tally up points or use a calorie counter. Simply don't eat if you're not hungry – and that means fat too.

- Never really getting into ketosis. Second, to eating too much protein, this is the most serious beginner mistake. If you can afford it and you're committed to the diet, get a ketosis meter. That way you'll know you're in the Goldilocks range of 1.5-3.0 mmol/L.

- Taking too many cheat days. If you decide to approach this diet with cheat days, don't do it unless you can limit the number of cheat days to two or fewer per month and you're sure you'll stick to it. Like everything else, it's good to track your cheat days in a journal or diary so that you KNOW where you stand. This will help you avoid major mistakes like taking two, then three, and then four cheat days in a month and finding out you haven't lost any weight.

Keto Foods and How They Affect the Body

Keto foods - provided that the amount of protein they contain is within the daily limits you're allowed – help you go into ketosis! We already know what the effects of ketosis are, so it's no mystery how keto foods impact the body. Keto foods will help you burn ketones instead of glucose. As a result, they can lead to rapid weight loss and all the other practical effects of ketosis we've already discussed.

Prohibited Foods

The list of prohibited foods on keto is long, but luckily, it's very easy to follow.

- Bread: Avoid all forms of bread, including whole grains. Simply put, on keto, you aren't going to eat bread. There are some commercially available low carb bread available, but they tend to be lacking. A good rule of thumb is to avoid bread all together for the first month or two and put wheat-based bread on the do not consume list. After you've been on keto for a while, search online for low carb breads that are made from substances like almond flour. But even then, make sure you know the exact number of carbs per serving.

- Pizza. We can qualify this one. If you can make a low carb crust and eat your pizza without going over 30 grams of carbohydrate per day, then you can eat pizza. But remember it can be full of hidden carbs in many places –

like tomato sauce. Be sure to count accurately. Regular pizza from a store is strictly prohibited.

- Fruit juices. People think of orange juice, or apple juice is healthy, but the reality is they are some of the worst foods you can consume. Don't drink fruit juice.

- Sodas, both diet and regular.

- Beer, in most cases.
- Root vegetables. A good rule of thumb to follow is that if a vegetable grows underground, you can't eat it. This includes carrots, turnips, potatoes, and sweet potatoes. Root vegetables are loaded with carbohydrates.

- Berries. Well actually you can consume berries, but in moderation and be sure to count the carbohydrates accurately. The best berries are the ones that are lowest in net sugar, including strawberries, blackberries, and raspberries. Blueberries are acceptable in smaller quantities, but they have more carbs than those already mentioned.

- Fruits. Think of a fruit as a natural sugar factory. Despite claims that they are necessary for health, you don't want to eat fruit on a keto diet. The lone exception is the avocado. Peaches might be one exception of a sugary fruit you can have in moderation.

- Pasta. Think of pasta like bread. Pasta is loaded with carbohydrates. A small serving would wreck your entire days' carbohydrate limits. It doesn't matter if its whole grain or not – don't eat pasta.

- Rice. Don't eat rice, even wild rice, and brown rice.

- Beans and legumes. While beans are a high protein food that is fiber-rich, they still contain too many carbohydrates for a keto diet. This is one reason why a vegetarian lifestyle isn't very compatible with keto.

- Sugar.

Beverages: What Is OK to Drink and What to Avoid

The simplest rule to follow is to drink water. However, it's possible to incorporate some other beverages into your keto lifestyle. Alcohol is a special case that we'll consider in the next chapter.

Don't drink sodas. And that means diet soda as well. You want to stay as natural as possible, and scientific research has shown that even diet sodas can cause weight gain. It's not entirely clear why that's the case, but the odds are that this type of phenomenon is going to be worse on keto. But one important aspect of soda including diet soda is how it's going to impact your fluid balance and hydration levels. We'll avoid mystery – the impacts are negative. You'll have to drink a lot of water to get back into balance after drinking a diet soda. It's best to avoid them simply.

Coffee and tea are permitted, but remember that they're diuretics. It does without saying you won't add sugar to your coffee or tea. Half and half should be avoided because although it's considered "fatty," it's watered down leaving a higher carb content. Use heavy cream instead, but don't use it in unlimited amounts. Cream has a small number of carbohydrates in it.

Something to consider is using butter in your coffee. A British cardiologist has recommended this.

Finally, avoid all "processed" drinks like red bull and other energy drinks.

Sugar and Artificial Sweeteners

Sugar is to be avoided at all costs. Calories and carbohydrates from sugar can add up quickly. If you put two teaspoons of sugar into a cup of tea, that's nearly 10 grams of carbs. If you're just starting and limiting yourself to 20 grams of carbs per day, that means you've already reached 50% of your daily limit. So, it's a good idea just to avoid it. Brown sugar is also to be avoided.

Opinions vary on artificial sweeteners. As far as safety, the reality is artificial sweeteners are safe. Any studies showing they can cause cancer have used absurd amounts. In a study that showed mice got cancer from Splenda, the mice were fed a diet equivalent to a human consuming 12,000 packs of Splenda per day. At that level, it's probably the case that anything causes cancer. Even water can kill you if you drink a massive amount over a short period.

The best advice to follow with artificial sweeteners is to consume in moderation. You can add two packs of Splenda or other artificial sweeteners to your coffee without having much impact on your diet. Just don't overdo it.

Stevia and xylitol are also acceptable options but remember to consume in moderation.

Required Ratios of Macronutrients

The key to keto is low carb, moderate protein, and high fat. But what does that mean, exactly? Let's take a look.

First, we might formally define what a "macro" is. In short macros are the general classes of nutrients as protein, fat, carbohydrate. It's also possible to include fiber and water in macros, but we won't do that here. Our focus will be on the big three: protein, fat, and carbs.

The general rule you want to follow is:

- 60-75% of calories from fat.
- 15-30% of calories from protein.
- 5-10% of calories from carbs.

You don't have to match up exactly with each meal, which is why there are allowed ranges that will let you stay in ketosis. While this information is useful, it's often easier to simply follow these rules:

- Eat a maximum of 30 grams of carbohydrate per day. Try to limit intake to 20 grams most days.
- Eat an amount of protein proportional to your body weight as we've already discussed. If you eat a half a gram of protein per pound of body weight per day, you won't have to struggle to worry about macronutrients.

Types of Fats: Good and Bad Fats

By now you've heard about bad fats. You've probably been brainwashed about bad fats nearly your entire life! The good news is that there really aren't many bad fats.

The good fats are natural, wholesome fats that include the following:

- *Monounsaturated fat.* The best sources are olive oil, avocado oil, or just eating avocados. Peanut oil is also a good fat.

- *Omega-3 oils.* These are the heart-healthy oils found in fatty fish. There are much fish you can eat on keto; the best are high-fat fish like salmon, sardines, anchovies, swordfish, and mackerel.

- *MCT oils.* The primary source of MCT fats is coconut oil. When you become more knowledgeable about the keto diet, you might be able to use MCT oils to increase your protein intake while still remaining in ketosis. Palm oils also contain MCTs and add a lot of interesting flavor to foods.

- *Saturated fats.* Yes, the devil has arrived. Doctors and nutritionists have unfairly demonized saturated fats for decades, but recent research has shown that it was all unjustified. The fact is if you're not eating a lot of carbs consuming saturated fats is just fine. Consider adding more butter to your diet.

There is only one real bad fat, and that's artificially manufactured trans-fats. This type of fat has been used for deep frying and in processed foods for decades. There is no doubt about the fact that artificial trans-fats are not good for you and raise your risk of heart disease. Of course, it's not like a molecule of the plague, one gram of trans-fats here and there is not going to send you to an early grave. But consuming them regularly can raise bad cholesterol and triglycerides while lowering your good cholesterol.

It's important to note that there are natural trans-fats. You will find these in some beef products. These should not be confused with artificially produced varieties, and there isn't any evidence that they cause health problems.

Finally, we come to vegetable oils. Some would classify them as bad fats, and if consumed in large amounts that's a fair characterization. In moderation, however, they aren't necessarily bad for you, but on a keto diet, they should be avoided. You should cook with olive oil or butter, and avoid fats like corn oil, canola oil, sunflower oil, and other similar omega-6 based oils.

The Role of Carbs in a Ketogenic Diet

Simply put when it comes to carbs you want to avoid them. The reality is the body doesn't need carbs to function; you can get by quite well on proteins and fats. However, you're going to want some carbohydrates, and in particular you're going to want those that aren't digestible. We call those kinds of carbohydrates *dietary fiber*.

An adequate amount of dietary fiber helps the body's digestive system function properly. This starts with your stomach and your small intestine and continues through the colon. A proper amount of dietary fiber will help you avoid appendicitis and helps the gall bladder perform its functions properly. Many people who are suffering from gall bladder disease may need to look at their fiber intake.

When it comes to the keto diet, two plant sources of food come to mind that are useful in not only providing needed minerals, but in providing adequate amounts of dietary fiber. The two foods we have in mind are celery and avocados. Both of these foods can be eaten in liberal quantities. Avocados, in particular, are a fantastic keto food because they are primarily a monounsaturated fat and dietary fiber. These foods will also help prevent constipation.

A second role of carbohydrates in the diet is simply as a vehicle to obtain needed antioxidants, vitamins, and minerals. Foods like spinach are packed with important minerals like potassium and magnesium, and also contain essential substances like vitamin K. Spinach contains minimal carbohydrates but does contain some, but you're not eating spinach with your steak to get energy, despite old myths. You're eating it to get the phytonutrients.

Beyond the two purposes laid out here, you don't need carbohydrates unless you have a specific health problem like type 1 diabetes. Most people can restrict their daily intake to 20 grams of carbs for very long periods – if not indefinitely – without any impact whatsoever.

Fats and proteins

When it comes to the ketogenic diet, think of fats as your energy source and proteins as a structural component. Proteins are vital for the body. People typically think of proteins as muscle – and that's one valuable role they play in the body. To avoid muscle loss with keto you'll need to be sure to get adequate protein intake as part of your diet. For most people, a protein intake of about 0.5 – 1.0 grams/pound is the right range. Don't go below

0.45 grams/pound, and always adjust your intake as you lose weight.

Keep in mind that protein isn't just about muscle mass; protein plays essential roles in the basic functioning of your body systems. For example, enzymes, which help drive the chemical reactions necessary for life, are made out of proteins. So, it's important to get adequate protein intake.

The problem with excess protein on a keto diet is that the body will use that as an excuse to make glucose. The liver can turn protein into glucose through a process known as *gluconeogenesis*. The details aren't necessary, all you need to know is that the body prefers using glucose because it's an easy energy source, and if you provide a backdoor way for the body to make glucose it's going to do it. The way that it does is by making it out of protein, and when that happens people find themselves unable to lose weight because their blood sugars are higher than they need to be.

Keeping an eye on ketones and blood sugar

Earlier we discussed a ketone meter. While it's not necessary, the best thing to do on a keto diet is to get a ketone meter and a blood glucose monitor so you know what your values are. You'll want to get baseline measurements before starting on your diet. In particular, you'll want to know your fasting blood sugar. Unless you're diabetic, it's not necessary to track your blood sugar daily, but once a week measurement to track your progress is a good idea. If you're starting with elevated blood sugars, obviously you'll want to know if keto is helping to get your blood sugar levels under control.

As we discussed earlier, you'll use a ketone meter to find out if you're actually in ketosis and how well it's going for you. Check to see if you're in the 1.5 mmol/l to 3.0 mmol/L range. If not, then take a look at what you ate that day and see if there are adjustments to be made.

As always, keep a journal or record of your numbers so you can accurately track your progress.

Best Times to Eat

Americans tend to make two major mistakes when it comes to eating no matter what kind of diet you're on. The first is skipping breakfast. We all get in a rush but skipping breakfast is a bad idea generally.

The second error people make is eating a large meal late at night. Does it make sense to consume a lot of calories and then watch TV for a while and go to sleep? It makes more sense to consume the bulk of your calories when you're more active. Eating your big meal earlier in the day is better. In Mediterranean cultures, the big meal of the day is consumed between 1 PM – 3 PM. Consider eating a larger meal earlier in the day at lunchtime and then enjoying a smaller dinner.

This isn't strictly necessary of course, and many people are simply too busy to prepare and eat a large meal at lunch. Many don't have time to eat a large meal at lunch. However, if you're going to eat your largest meal at night, its best to eat it earlier in the evening rather than later, and you'll want to avoid eating a large meal close to bedtime.

There are options available for keto dieters who are pressed for time. Go on Amazon or to a local health food store and look for keto drink mixer options. There are many excellent mixes made for keto shakes that you can use. Some are quite tasty and satisfying, being made out of interesting foods like dried and powdered butter. Be sure to check the details and ensure that the shake is really keto friendly. Do this by checking the macronutrients. You may also consider what the shake is made out of including the protein source. Some will want whey protein, but others might prefer avoiding it.

You'll also want to give some thought about what kind of liquid you'll use if you decide to make shakes. Make sure you avoid carbs. Almond milk can be used as long as it's unsweetened. Don't use regular milk, even whole milk because it contains a large amount of carbohydrate.

Heavy cream can be used in place of milk for those looking for a high-calorie drink, but keep in mind that cream contains some carbohydrates. A cup of heavy cream contains nearly 7 grams of carbohydrate, so must be included when adding up your daily carbs. A cup of cream also contains 800 calories. While we don't count calories on keto, you do need to have some idea about it and don't want to go overboard.

Another suggestion is to mix a heavy fat like cream or even olive oil with unsweetened almond milk in your shake.

Customizing Keto

The keto diet isn't a rigid set of rules as long as you stay within the limits of ketosis. Some people will find that they can add more carbohydrates to their diet and still remain in keto, while others will have to take an approach that keeps carbs within very strict limits.

To make things interesting, you might look at other diets and find out if they can be turned into keto diets. One way to customize a keto diet is to only eat fish as your meat source, something that may work out for some.

Chapter 3: Keto and Weight Loss

We've discussed many of the benefits of a keto diet. Since the body uses ketones for fuel, the fat burning effect leads to weight loss. In many people, the weight loss will be fast and dramatic. At the beginning of the diet your body will burn a lot of glycogen, which is a form of the stored body in your muscle cells. The exciting thing about glycogen is that one glycogen molecule is bound to four water molecules. You may have heard that people on Atkins or keto lose a lot of "water weight." This is the reason that happens – your body burns up excess glycogen when faced with a new shortage of carbohydrate, and the water comes out with it. After this initial phase true and regular fat burning can begin. In this early phase, your body may go through unpleasant effects like the "keto flu" discussed earlier, but if you stick to it through this phase and make adjustments such as drinking the right amount of water and taking the right supplements, your body will adjust to such perceived maladies.

Generally speaking, people who have more body fat are going to do better on keto than people who start with relatively less weight to lose.

After the initial adjustment phase, your body is now used to being on keto. During this phase, you'll find you have better energy and mental clarity. Weight loss will be more gradual during this phase, but if you stay in ketosis, you can expect to continue losing a couple of pounds per week.

A ketogenic diet is going to be the most effective if you're one of those people who have trouble with carbohydrates. You don't have to be a diabetic either. Keto is going to result in massive weight loss for anyone who's been eating the standard American diet and steadily gaining weight over the years. But the fact is millions of people are literally being poisoned by having too many carbohydrates in their diet and aren't even aware of it.

Even if diabetes isn't something in your genes, the more you pile on the carbs in your diet the harder you're making your pancreas work. The body's cells become insulin resistant, meaning that they're less responsive to a given amount of insulin in the bloodstream. The result? More insulin is required to accomplish the same amount of work. For some people over time no amount of insulin gets the job done – those are the people who have diabetes or suffering from pre-diabetes. Other people still won't be pre-diabetes yet, but their cells are still forcing the pancreas to pump out more insulin to overcome the slowly increasing resistance. Over time this leads to more body fat, since one of the functions of insulin is to direct the body to store excess calories as body fat.

When you follow a keto lifestyle, this vicious cycle is eliminated. Instead of your body constantly battling excess sugars, it's burning fat for fuel instead. That means it will burn off your body fat and you'll start losing weight.

The biggest key with keto is people usually lose weight effortlessly. A dieter will find themselves eating fatty rib eye steaks, chicken with the skin on, avocadoes, and butter, and yet tipping the scale a little less each day. The results can come in shockingly rapid fashion. In this video, Jordan Peterson describes his weight loss – seven pounds a month for seven months in a row.

https://youtu.be/tw8Rf9ho-Sk

Most people will find they lose weight rapidly if they strictly follow a keto diet. And even those who only diet intermittently will also find they lose weight. However, you should make sure you follow the keto style of eating at least 3-4 days per week if you decide to go down that path.

Remember we said there were two caveats. The second caveat is to avoid eating too much protein. Failing to follow this rule sinks a lot of keto dieters. If you find yourself losing a lot of weight initially but then hit a plateau, consider your protein intake.

Chapter 4: Lowering Your Triglycerides

Triglycerides are a type of fat found in the blood, which are made every time you eat. While insulin will trigger the cells to take up the blood sugar they need for energy, any excess calories that have been consumed will be converted into triglycerides by the liver. Triglycerides are released into the bloodstream and then transported through the bloodstream. Triglycerides are then converted into stored fat on the body. Some people have defective liver metabolism and will produce more triglycerides than others given the same caloric and carb intake.

The biggest culprits when it comes to triglycerides are sugar and alcohol. If you consume alcohol to excess, you're probably going to raise your triglyceride levels. In fact, a problem alcoholics sometimes encounter is they increase their triglyceride levels to extremely high standards, triggering a life-threatening condition known as pancreatitis. The details aren't important here, but what happens is the pancreas works extra hard as a result of the high blood levels of triglycerides.

Fasting blood levels of triglycerides can be summarized by these categories:

- Very high: to reach this level your fasting triglyceride level would be 500 mg/dL or higher.
- High: this range is 200 to 499 mg/dL.
- Borderline: 150 to 199 mg/dL.
- Normal: Below 150 mg/dL.
- Ideal: Below 80 mg/dL.

If your triglyceride level (fasting) is borderline, your doctor is likely to advise limiting alcohol consumption and making dietary and exercise changes. Losing weight can also help lower fasting triglyceride numbers, although in some cases the cause is simple genetics or family history. If your fasting triglyceride number is high or very high, medication is likely to be prescribed.

Even if you're not an alcoholic, high triglyceride levels can put your body at risk for pancreatitis and other problems. Medical professionals consider a fasting triglyceride level of 150 or lower to be reasonable. A level below 100 is better, and 70 or below is ideal. If your fasting triglyceride level is above 200, your doctor may put you on a medication called gemfibrozil. Alternatively, triglyceride levels can be lowered with high consumption of EPA, a type of fish oil. Following this approach requires consuming at least 3,000 mg of EPA per day. While there is a prescription medication available that contains EPA, you can purchase purified EPA over the counter as well. If you decide to do so, you should make sure that you can readily get the required 3,000 mg per day of fish oil from the product. Also, be sure to consult with your doctor before consuming that much fish oil to make sure you don't have any pre-existing health problems that could lead to difficulties.

Pancreatitis isn't the only risk of high triglyceride levels. In fact, if you're not an alcoholic pancreatitis is relatively rare, except cases where the patient has bile duct problems. The main concern with high triglyceride levels is with heart disease.

We've discussed this earlier in the book. The primary dietary culprit besides alcohol consumption in high triglyceride numbers is the consumption of carbohydrates, in particular simple sugars. Many doctors will advise consuming "whole grains," but the reality is for lots of people whole gains will keep triglyceride levels elevated. Since triglyceride levels are directly related to the consumption of excess calories, it's easy to see why eating a lot of carbohydrates can raise triglyceride levels.

Your levels of triglycerides and HDL or "good" cholesterol are tied closely together. HDL means *high-density lipoprotein*. It's a type of cholesterol that actually cleans out the LDL or "bad" cholesterol from your arteries.

High triglycerides can lead to the development of heart disease. In fact, it's slowly being recognized as one of the most important factors. Type 2 diabetics in particular – and those not yet diabetic but potentially diabetic – tend to have high triglycerides. In short:

- High blood sugar levels often correspond to higher triglyceride levels and lower levels of HDL or "good" cholesterol.
- People with weight problems tend to have higher triglyceride levels.
- High triglyceride levels correspond to smaller, and denser LDL or "bad" cholesterol molecules.

Since triglycerides are transported through the bloodstream by LDL cholesterol, the fact that the body has a certain level of cholesterol it needs to transport using LDL means that crowding out by triglycerides translates into more LDL particles. Since triglycerides pack densely, this also means the particles are smaller, and so pose a greater risk of sticking to arterial walls, leading to heart disease.

Factors that influence triglyceride level include:

- Weight gain
- High fasting blood sugar levels
- More body fat
- Consumption of carbohydrates
- Alcohol
- High fasting blood sugars
- Lack of exercise

Of the factors on the list, exercise is the least important, and studies showing that exercise helps triglyceride levels might be since people who exercise are in better shape in general, having less body fat, healthier body weight, and lower blood sugar levels.

Lower HDL levels which are associated with high triglyceride and high blood sugar levels, cause problems as well. HDL or "good" cholesterol acts as a type of vacuum cleaner in the bloodstream, sucking up excess LDL molecules for transport back to the liver. By reducing LDL particle number, HDL reduces the probability that LDL molecules will stick to the arterial walls leading to heart disease. Low HDL values indicate you don't have enough HDL in your bloodstream to effectively "clean it out."

Factors that can increase HDL include:

- Losing weight.
- Exercise.
- Consumption of healthy fats like monounsaturated fats and omega-3 oils.

- Consumption of MCT fats, which are found in coconut and palm oil (be aware that coconut and palm oil also have high concentrations of saturated fats as well).
- Eating a low carbohydrate diet.

Since a ketogenic diet hits several of these points, dieters typically see their HDL increase.

We've seen that HDL level, blood sugar level, and triglyceride level are all related, but what's the connection? It turns out its insulin sensitivity. A good indirect way to measure insulin sensitivity is to check your triglyceride to HDL level. This is also a good measure of heart attack risk, as we've discussed previously. To calculate this level, you only need two pieces of data:

- Your fasting triglyceride number
- Your fasting HDL number

Then divide the triglyceride number by your HDL number. For example, suppose that Susan has a fasting triglyceride number of 180 mg/DL, and her fasting HDL value is 40 mg/dL. Then her triglyceride to HDL ratio is:

Ratio = triglycerides/HDL = 180/40 = 4.5

Any value above 3 is considered a high risk for heart disease. It also indicates that Susan has problems with insulin sensitivity, and her blood sugar is likely to be high as well. Note again that we are talking about fasting values. Note that when taken alone, even though Susan's HDL number might be considered low normal and her triglyceride level is only moderately elevated, when taken together these numbers tell us that Susan is in fact at *high risk* of heart disease. A ketogenic diet can definitely help someone like Susan, by lowering her triglyceride levels and possibly raising her HDL levels as well.

When you are insulin resistant, this means that you're producing enough insulin, but the cells are not responding properly and removing glucose from the blood. People who are insulin resistant are at higher risk of developing diabetes and may suffer from a condition called metabolic syndrome. In contrast, consider John, who has a fasting triglyceride level of 100 mg/dL and a fasting HDL value of 50 mg/dL. For John, we find a triglyceride to HDL level of:

Ratio = triglycerides/HDL = 100/50 = 2

His level is well below 3, so we consider John to be in a healthy range. He is considered at moderate risk for cardiovascular disease. However, even John could benefit from adopting a keto or low-carb diet because he could lower his triglyceride level even more. Consuming more fish can also help.

Even though the keto diet can massively improve your blood lipid numbers, it's important to exercise as well. In several large studies, it has been shown that moderate to vigorous physical activity significantly reduces the incidence of cardiovascular events such as heart attack and stroke. This has also been studied by comparing triglyceride to HDL ratios with the level of cardiovascular fitness. It has been found that levels of cardiovascular fitness and triglyceride to HDL ratios are *independent* predictors of future heart attack and stroke. Therefore, it's important to incorporate some exercise into your keto lifestyle and not rely entirely on the diet alone. It's not necessary to become a triathlete to get the benefits. You can achieve a healthy level of fitness by incorporating moderate exercise such as a daily 30-minute walk into your routine. Depending on your health status more may be required. Generally, 150 minutes of walking per week is considered to be the required level of moderate activity that will reduce cardiovascular risk. If you are engaging in more vigorous exercise, such as jogging or bicycling, the time required is lower. It's generally accepted that about half the weekly effort is necessary when pursuing vigorous exercise, so those doing so should shoot for about 75 minutes per week of activity.

Chapter 5: Normalize Your Blood Sugar

By now you've probably figured out that several risk factors for heart disease go hand-in-hand. This is known as "risk factor clustering." The risk factors for the development of heart disease that often come together in the same individuals includes (fasting values):

- Low HDL cholesterol
- High triglyceride levels
- High blood sugar levels (often high enough to be diagnosed with pre-diabetes)
- Obesity
- Low insulin sensitivity
- High blood pressure

When a person has all of these risk factors, it's called metabolic syndrome. The focal point of all of these problems tends to be high blood sugar – something that is the result of *low insulin sensitivity.*

The Impact of Keto on Insulin

A keto diet has positive impacts on insulin. Low carbohydrate consumption translates to lower levels of insulin in the body because more insulin isn't necessary. Even when not eating, the effects are felt. Keto dieters have lower levels of fasting insulin than do people that consume carbohydrates. Simply put when you have less sugar to deal with your body makes less insulin. A keto diet will lower fasting insulin levels, stabilize blood sugar, and improve insulin sensitivity. What this means is that when the body does need to use insulin, it will work more efficiently.

You can try to address insulin sensitivity by taking medications such as metformin, or you can address it naturally by changing your diet. Keto diet helps address insulin sensitivity by reducing the number of carbohydrates consumed. A natural extension of this is that fasting blood sugar levels are naturally reduced leading to a healthier overall state of the body.

A beginner's mistake often made on ketogenic diets is that people starting the ketogenic diet aren't really eating keto. This happens when people eat too much protein. When excess amounts of protein are consumed, if there are not also a lot of carbohydrates in the diet your liver will make glucose out of the protein. For this reason, it's important to maintain an adequate but moderate level of protein in your daily diet. This is done by keeping protein consumption at a level of 0.45 to 0.5 grams per pound of body weight.

For example, when Steve starts his ketogenic diet, he weighs 200 pounds. So he should consume:

- At least 90 grams of protein per day. We arrive at this number using 0.45 grams/pound * 200 pounds = 90 grams of protein.
- At most 100 grams of protein per day. We arrive at this number using 0.5 grams/pound * 200 pounds = 100 grams of protein.

It's just as important to consume an adequate amount of protein as it is to avoid consuming excess protein. If you fail to consume enough protein, then you might find yourself losing muscle tissue and not just fat. We certainly don't want to lose weight by losing muscle mass.

When Steve loses some weight, he will need to reduce his protein consumption. Let's suppose that after a week Steve has lost ten pounds. Now he weighs 190 pounds and he should adjust his protein consumption accordingly:

- At least 85.5 grams of protein per day. We arrive at this number using 0.45 grams/pound * 190 pounds = 85.5 grams of protein.
- At most 95 grams of protein per day. We arrive at this number using 0.45 grams/pound * 190 pounds = 95 grams of protein.

The takeaways are that burning ketones instead of sugar will result in lower fasting blood sugars and help deal with metabolic syndrome. By consuming the right level of proteins we ensure that we won't have hidden sources of blood sugar in our diets.

Chapter 6: Alcohol and Keto

The consumption of alcohol is something that has to be carefully considered while on the keto diet. Many people aren't aware of this, but when you're on keto and making your liver work by turning fats into usable ketone bodies, it's going to be harder for your liver to process alcohol too. That means that some people are going to have a hard time drinking while they are in ketosis. You might find yourself getting intoxicated after consuming a much smaller amount of alcohol than you're used to.

If you run into this sort of problem, you'll want to step back and figure out if drinking alcohol is all that important to you. If you decide that you want to keep drinking, you'll have to adjust your behavior accordingly. This means determining what your new limits are and even considering going off ketosis before drinking, as long as that's not a frequent occurrence. If it's something you're going to do just once in a while, you can consume a small meal of a carbohydrate-rich food before drinking alcohol. Doing so will get the liver off the hook when dealing with ketones so it will be freed up to deal with the onslaught of alcohol.

Alcohol can be consumed in moderation, but drinking too much can cause problems when it comes to losing weight, even on keto. The body will burn alcohol before it burns other fuels, so if you drink too much in one sitting, you'll find yourself not losing weight as expected. The best thing to do if you decide to drink while on keto is to follow the general advice on drinking in moderation. Using wine as an example, stick to 1-2 glasses per day for women and 2-3 glasses per day with men. Also, be aware that you'll have to know how many carbs are in the alcohol you're drinking and include it in your daily totals.

ɔhol that should be avoided include beer and sugary
s. Hard liquor and other spirits, as well as wine and
make better options for keto dieters.

Once you've determined your limits, the next thing to do is
familiarize yourself with the carb content of alcoholic drinks to
determine which ones are suitable to use with keto. Let's start
with the most frequently consumed drinks, beer, and wine.
Obviously, details vary, but we'll use average carb loads per
serving:

- Beer: 10-13 carbs (per 12 oz. serving).
- Red wine: 2 carbs (standard wine glass, 5 oz.).
- White wine: 2 carbs (standard wine glass, 5 oz.).
- Champagne: 1-2 carbs (5 oz. serving).

Be aware that sweeter tasting wines will have higher
carbohydrate levels than those cited here. A typical sweet wine
such as a Riesling will contain twice as many carbs or about 4
per glass. Dry wines are preferred on a keto diet.

An interesting aside is that wine is a nutritious drink. One glass
of merlot, for example, contains 187 mg of potassium, 5% of the
recommended daily allowance of vitamin B-6, and 4% of the
recommended daily allowance of magnesium. Of course, it's not
a good idea to be drinking wine to get your potassium, but it's
good to know that you're getting more out of it than alcohol.

Beer is another story. If you're on a ketogenic diet, then beer is
something you'll want to avoid. People tend to think of beer as
starchy, and that's an accurate perception, as is the term "beer
belly." It's pretty clear that if you're on a keto diet and limiting

your daily carb intake to 20-30 grams per day, a "couple of beers" are going to wreck your diet totally.

Craft beers and varieties like IPA are even worse. A 12-ounce Sierra Nevada IPA contains 175 calories and 14 grams of carbs. Many IPAs have even more carbs, some up to 20 grams per serving. Making things even worse is the fact that if you go out somewhere, chances are you're not going to be getting a 12-ounce serving. Most places will serve beer in pints or 22-ounce sizes. This means that drinking beer adds a lot of carbohydrates to your daily intake.

Hard drinks or so-called "spirits" offer low or zero carb options. Soda water (unsweetened) can be used to make a low carb mixed drink. Some *zero* carb options include:

- Whiskey
- Tequila
- Vodka
- Dry martini
- Brandy

Mixed drinks are more problematic and need to be chosen with care. Many contain sugary syrups and carbohydrates as the main ingredient. A margarita contains 8 carbs per serving while a white Russian contains around 17. A bloody Mary checks in at around 7 carbs per serving. Adding orange juice or sugary sodas to your drink can create a high sugar drink with a large number of carbs double or more these values, so it's probably best to avoid them. Mixed drinks that only use carbonated sodas and lime or lemon (for example) are usually low carb and make good substitutes.

Chapter 7: Cholesterol and Keto

One of the major objections raised with keto is that it will raise your cholesterol. For many people it will raise it, but it's important to look at the details. Doctors used to look only at the total cholesterol number, but have since discovered there are different types and subtypes of cholesterol. When it comes to keto, it's important to understand what they are and know their values to make sense out of your numbers.

Cholesterol is basically a kind of fatty material. Since fat and water don't mix, the body packages cholesterol with a type of protein so that it can be transported through the blood. The bound molecules are called a *lipoprotein*, meaning fat + protein. The proteins that are a part of cholesterol help move it through the blood to where it needs to go in the body. Cholesterol is a very useful substance, it's used to help build cell membranes and to manufacture important hormones in the body like vitamin-d and testosterone. People who have very low levels of "bad" cholesterol are actually at higher risk of death from all causes. Your body needs "bad" cholesterol, you don't want too much and having it stick to the walls of your arteries, clogging up the pipes and doing damage.

By now everyone has heard about *good* and *bad* cholesterol. Good cholesterol is called HDL. HDL means "high-density lipoprotein," and it's called "good" cholesterol because its function in the body is to remove the LDL or "bad" cholesterol from your bloodstream. This helps protect against the buildup of plaque in your arteries.

A high HDL number means a lower long-term risk of heart disease. For most people, following a keto lifestyle will raise your

HDL number. It turns out that several blood markers – HDL, triglycerides, and blood sugar – tend to be related in how they move in response to diet. While not true in all cases, for most people weight gain and problems maintaining healthy blood sugar levels correspond to lower HDL numbers and higher triglyceride numbers. This is fixed by going into ketosis, and the best way to do that is to eat a ketogenic diet. To summarize:

A higher HDL number means a lower risk of heart disease, and most people will see their HDL number go up while following a keto diet.

LDL stands for low-density lipoprotein, and it's known as "bad" cholesterol because more LDL translates into a higher risk of heart disease – generally speaking. When doctors talk about high cholesterol numbers, they are talking about the LDL number, and most blood tests now give a specific measurement for LDL.

However, it turns out that just knowing your LDL number doesn't tell the whole story. The size of LDL particles is also important. Smaller LDL particles are more likely to stick to your artery walls and cause cardiovascular disease. A ketogenic diet will make LDL particles larger, while a diet high in carbohydrates tends to make them smaller.

- A ketogenic diet makes LDL or "bad" cholesterol molecules light and fluffy. They can travel through the blood stream without doing much damage.
- A diet high in carbohydrates, especially a sugar-laden diet, will make LDL particles small and hard, making them more likely to stick to artery walls and cause cardiovascular disease.

These two facts explain a lot. In particular, it describes why saturated fat has been associated with heart disease in the past. Saturated fat is made into LDL cholesterol by the liver. So eating more saturated fat from beef or chicken skin can raise your LDL number. Now we see where the confusion comes in. If you're eating a lot of saturated fat *and* following a high carbohydrate diet, your LDL number will go up, and the LDL particles will be hard, small, and sticky – leading to heart disease.

However, if you are following a low carb diet, especially a keto diet, the saturated fat you consume is going to be packaged by the liver into light and fluffy LDL particles that travel through the blood stream without sticking to your arterial walls and causing heart disease. You can summarize this by saying it's not the beef patty that causes heart disease in the typical American diet, it's *the beef patty together with the French fries and bun* that cause heart disease.

- A diet that is high in carbohydrates should limit saturated fat to keep LDL cholesterol lower. The combination of saturated fat + carbohydrates tends to produce smaller and dangerous LDL particles. Doctors typically recommend limiting saturated fat to 20 grams or less if you are eating a normal diet with a high number of carbohydrates.
- A diet that is low in carbohydrates can be high in saturated fat because the LDL particles will be light and fluffy, and heart disease does not develop. On the keto diet you can eat saturated fat without worrying about it.

Now we learn that triglycerides play a role here too. LDL particles carry triglycerides with them, and the more triglycerides they carry the fewer cholesterol molecules they

68

carry. Think of it as an airplane with a fixed number of seats, and people are wearing green suits or white suits. Let's also suppose that the people in green suits were going on optional flights, but the people in white suits were going on required flights.

The more people are wearing green suits (triglycerides) that board the plane, the fewer people wearing white suits (cholesterol) that can board the plane. So to transport all the people in white suits to their destinations, the more airplanes you need. On the other hand, if there were fewer people in green suits, more people with white suits could board the airplane and you'd have fewer airplanes and fewer flights.

That is one reason why high triglycerides raise the risk of heart disease. They take up space in your LDL particles, and so the body needs more LDL particles to transport cholesterol. It also affects the density of the LDL particles. You can think of them as small and hard. Small and hard LDL particles stick to artery walls and cause heart disease.

Conversely, if you have lower levels of triglycerides, there is more room for cholesterol in an LDL particle. So a given LDL particle packs more cholesterol in it, and it's going to be larger in size, light and fluffy. LDL particles that are light and fluffy don't stick to artery walls and don't raise heart disease risk.

These observations explain a lot, including why a keto diet is healthy and effective. One of the most important effects of the keto diet is to lower triglycerides. So while an increased consumption of fats, saturated fat in particular, may raise total cholesterol in some people and total LDL cholesterol, it does not mean your heart disease risk has increased. You can have your doctor track your LDL-P number (where P is for particle number) as well as the LDL number, so you can learn how your particle number is progressing. A higher cholesterol number with a lower LDL-P means you're in a healthier state. So let's summarize the impact of keto on cholesterol:

- Following a keto diet lowers triglycerides.
- A keto diet tends to increase HDL.
- More HDL means that LDL or bad cholesterol is cleaned out from the bloodstream more effectively; lowering the risk you'll develop plaque.
- A lower triglyceride number means that you'll have fewer LDL particles, each of which carries more cholesterol per particle. They will be larger, and "fluffy" and not stick to arterial walls, so don't raise the risk of heart disease.

If you're not able to get a detailed LDL profile with your blood lipid tests, you can simply use triglycerides as a proxy. A level below 150 is the standard value considered healthy by the medical establishment. Many on a keto diet will see their triglyceride level drop below 100 and even into the range of 50-60.

Finally, remember to track your triglyceride to HDL value. Get your triglyceride number and divide it by the HDL number to get the ratio.

- If your triglyceride to HDL ratio is 3 or more, you're at higher risk of heart disease.
- If your triglyceride to HDL ratio is less than 3, you're at decreased risk of heart disease.

As discussed above, the keto diet is likely to cause the following changes to your cholesterol panel:

- Your HDL cholesterol will rise.
- Your LDL cholesterol may rise, causing total cholesterol to rise.
- However, your LDL-P number will decrease, indicating better health.
- Your triglyceride levels will decrease.

Why High Total Cholesterol Isn't Necessarily Bad

As discussed above, high total cholesterol isn't necessarily bad. When you go on a keto diet your triglyceride levels will decrease, and HDL may increase. So, if you're total cholesterol an increase, this likely reflects that your HDL level has increased. Moreover, your LDL level has probably increased as well, but the type of LDL molecules is more important than the raw number. If possible, find out how your LDL-P number is changing with time. A keto diet likely means that you're going to have larger and less damaging LDL particles and there will be fewer in number, even though the raw cholesterol number may be higher. The best metric you should keep track of is the triglyceride to HDL value. A lower value indicates a healthier LDL.

Earlier we discussed a ketone meter, it's also possible to buy a home meter that checks your cholesterol, HDL, and triglyceride levels. You will have to infer your overall LDL cholesterol number as this test is not available with existing home meters. An excellent meter to look at is called *Cardiochek*. You can find out your triglyceride and HDL numbers and track your ratios. Be sure to only test fasting values, and go 8-12 hours without eating before doing the test. The device is FDA approved, but you may want to repeat tests and average because the error rate will be higher than that seen with a test done at the doctor's office, with a larger amount of blood.

Chapter 8: Incorporating Exercise into a Keto Lifestyle

The main issue with exercise and keto is that at first, your body enters a transition period where you might experience low energy levels and brain "fog." Deprived of glucose, your body has to adjust to making and using ketone bodies for energy. For some people this is not a problem, while others will have to adjust to the "keto flu." The good news is that this will pass once your body becomes fully adjusted and your energy levels will increase.

If you suffer from this issue, you shouldn't stop exercising, but you probably won't want to hit it hard or add new challenges to your exercise routine either. The key to exercise and keto is consuming enough fat.

Once you transition to keto fat is your energy source, so it's important that you genuinely consume the levels of fat the diet demands. If you eat enough fat, then you'll have enough energy for your workouts and find that you burn more fat off your body when you do exercise.

Some recent research into the benefits of exercise has uncovered surprises that might be to the liking of most readers. Previously, it had been thought that to attain cardiovascular fitness a person had to engage in 20 or 30 minutes of "vigorous" exercise per day to get the benefits. When researchers studied people who were regular runners, however, they came across a stunning result – people who only ran five minutes a day got most of the health benefits that those running 30 minutes or an hour got from their running. The runners were followed over a long time period, and it was found that all runners had a lower risk of death and cardiovascular disease as compared to people who didn't exercise, or did so at moderate levels. But the differences between those who ran only five minutes and those running for long time periods wasn't really all that significant. You can find a nice lay person's discussion of this research in the New York Times.

So it appears that people get the majority of the benefit that hard cardiovascular training provides after only a short period of exercising.

This surprising result provides an alternative for people who aren't very excited about putting in long days at the gym. It may be possible that you can get the same benefits by just going on a short jog.

Now we aren't giving out specific health advice in this book, so it's up to each individual to do the research and find out what works best for him or her. One possible way to rev up your exercise without having to kill yourself is to do a 30-minute walk three or four days a week, and do a five-minute jog three days a week. That way you're getting a little bit of both.

At the time of writing, researchers aren't sure if the five-minute benefits accrue to other types of exercise. So they aren't sure if riding on an exercise bike for five minutes a day will provide the same benefits or not, but common sense seems to imply that it would if you use a good level of intensity.

In any case, when it comes down to exercise, you need to tailor it both to your own needs and also to something you like doing. Enjoyment of exercise is directly proportional to how much you do and whether or not you stick to it.

It's important to note that on a keto lifestyle, exercise is not strictly required. Simply following a keto diet will enable you to lose weight and do so rapidly and consistently, provided that you're strictly following the guidelines. However, for optimal health cardiovascular exercise is recommended. In large-scale studies that have tracked people for blood markers like triglycerides, HDL cholesterol, and total cholesterol, as well as tracking their exercise habits, it has been found that those who exercised and managed their blood lipids were at the lowest risk of heart attack and stroke.

Those who exercised but didn't maintain good blood lipids had lower cardiovascular risk than people who didn't exercise at all, but had higher cardiovascular risk than people who exercised and had good blood lipids. Conversely, those who had good blood lipid profiles had lower cardiovascular risk than the general population. However, if they didn't exercise, they had a higher risk than those who exercised and had good blood lipids.

What are we saying here? The bottom line is that having good blood lipids, as defined by low triglycerides, low LDL or "bad" cholesterol, and high HDL, as well as low blood sugar is very important. And you'll get this profile by following a keto diet carefully.

However, people who do this *and* exercise are at the lowest risk.

The goal of exercising should be to obtain a minimal level of cardiovascular fitness. It's not the time spent exercising or what you do that appears to be important, but whether you've conditioned your body in such a way that you can withstand the challenge that says a five-minute run entails.

If you don't exercise at all, a five-minute run might be extremely challenging. Many middle-aged or older people who don't engage in regular exercise will be able to run *even that much.* That's why a five-minute jog is probably connected to significantly lower risks of heart attack and stroke – because that small amount of time commitment is enough to condition the body.

Believe it or not, some recent research has taken this concept even further. Some researchers have found that a one or two minutes of aerobic exercise appears to condition people's bodies well enough that cardiovascular disease risk is significantly reduced. What we're talking about here is running all-out sprints for at least one minute, as hard and fast as you can run.

Exercising just a minute a day might sound very appealing – and it might work out for you. But, If you have an underlying heart problem and run at an all-out sprint, it might be enough to trigger a heart attack.

We should also mention that cardiovascular disease isn't the only risk factor that short bouts of exercise appear to impact. They also appear to reduce the risk of death from all causes.

Chapter 9: Keto and Insomnia

Lack of sleep is a significant health problem, leading to obesity, overeating, hormone changes and other health problems. If you don't get good nights sleep, you'll have trouble making it through the day and mentally focusing.

For some people, keto may cause insomnia problems in the early stages of the diet. In most cases, this is driven by the "keto flu." The odds are that it will pass once your body fully adjusts and you're burning ketones for fuel. The key here is the same as it is with exercise – make sure you're getting enough fat in your diet. If you're feeling low energy and not getting good nights sleep, consider increasing your fat intake.

Conversely, you might be getting more energy from fat. That is keto is working out really well for you, but you're so energetic that going to sleep is more difficult. In that case, try eating your last meal earlier in the evening.

Another problem that causes insomnia on keto is depletion of your glycogen stores. Glycogen is sugar stored in your muscle cells. Each glycogen molecule is bound to four molecules of water. People who need to lose weight not only have extra fat they're carrying around, they also have higher glycogen stores on average.

When you start the keto diet one of the things that happen is your body rapidly uses up its excess storage of glycogen, to keep burning sugars for fuel. This is a good thing – you'll be healthier once you're rid of this excess. But an unpleasant side effect of this is that you'll probably be urinating more than you're used to as the body gets rid of the water that has been stored with the glycogen. This is the proverbial 'water weight' problem.

So what happens when you have to pee a lot more? You might find yourself having to go more at night, and getting up frequently to go to the bathroom can cause insomnia problems. The good news is that this problem will pass in a short period once your glycogen stores become adjusted to a reasonable level.

The final factor that can lead to insomnia problems on a keto diet is an improper electrolyte balance. We've seen this problem rear its ugly head before in other areas. So make sure that you're not just focused on fat and meat – get your minerals. Try drinking a cup of broth every day and make sure you're also getting adequate potassium and magnesium to keep your sodium in balance. You can take magnesium supplements, but great sources of potassium and magnesium include leafy greens like spinach, broccoli, and avocados, which also contain large amounts of healthful monounsaturated fat. When eaten in moderation, macadamia nuts can also help provide needed minerals and monounsaturated fats, but they shouldn't be consumed until you've been on the diet for a few weeks. Also, keep track of any carbs you consume from nuts.

Chapter 10: Keto and Acne

A surprising benefit of the keto diet is that in some people, keto will decrease and even cure acne problems. Over the past few decades, people didn't connect acne with diet because research had failed to link high levels of acne to specific foods. However, the problem was they weren't looking at macros, and during most of the research period people weren't interested in a keto diet.

It turns out that acne is related to hormonal imbalances. In your skin, sebaceous glands produce oils that keep your skin lubricated. In people with serious acne problems, this process is disrupted.

Elevated androgens cause the production of a compound called *sebum* in the skin as well as make the skin more oily. Sebum can clog skin pores, which also traps bacteria that were on your skin. A small infection results and you develop a pimple, which is simply the body's attempt to trap, isolate and get rid of an infection. In short, acne is an inflammatory response. Androgens are "male" hormones, and more of them are produced in adolescence and young adulthood, which is why teenagers are more likely to produce acne. Many adults have problems with acne as well.

And guess what can exacerbate these types of hormonal imbalances? A high level of carbohydrate consumption. Keto immediately fixes this problem and so many people on keto find that their acne has been substantially reduced.

In the early stages of the diet, however, you might find your acne worsening. You can relax about this knowing that like other effects this is likely to be temporary. People more prone to issues like keto flu may also have temporarily worsening acne. As the body adjusts to burning fat and depleting excess glycogen stores, it's also going to adjust proper hormone levels that can impact acne. If you're in this situation give it a short amount of time. Over time a keto diet – followed closely without cheating – will lead to clearer skin.

There are several reasons for this. Remember that a keto diet will result in lower insulin levels. It turns out that high insulin levels also contribute to more oils and sebum in the skin, raising the risk of acne problems. The second factor that contributes to reducing acne is that keto diets reduce inflammation overall. Remember that acne is an inflammatory response. When you have less inflammation, you're less likely to develop acne.

Finally, a special hormone called *insulin-like growth factor-1* or IGF-1 has been shown to increase the propensity to develop acne. It turns out that ketogenic diets will reduce levels of IGF-1 in the body, and therefore reduce the propensity to develop acne.

Chapter 11: Keto and Stress

It can be said that a ketogenic diet is an elixir for mental health. There have been hints of this for centuries since it was known that keto diets helped control epilepsy in children. But it has taken a long time to connect the benefits of keto to other brain functions, including mental clarity and better mental health.

High blood sugars cause stress at the cellular level and with this comes the release of stress hormones like cortisol. This causes feelings of stress and inflammation throughout the body. The result is you feel more stress and anxiety in your mental states.
By reducing carbohydrates, the level of stress at the cellular level and beyond is also reduced. Stress hormones like cortisol are released in smaller amounts, and this creates a better mental perception.

People on keto will find that they have lower rates of anxiety, sleep better, and have lower perceptions of stress overall. But keep in mind that once again, the "keto flu" phenomena might influence your early experiences on the keto diet. That means initially you might find your stress and anxiety levels increase – but like other aspects of keto flu, this is temporary.

The keto diet addresses stress and anxiety primarily by regulating hormones. High blood sugars can wreak havoc by causing stress that leads your adrenal glands to release various hormones. This problem is made worse in people that have even moderate difficulties with blood sugar, in particular with blood sugar "spikes." Even ordinary people have blood sugar spikes – if you eat a meal with a large component of carbohydrates about two hours after eating your blood sugar will spike.

In a supposedly healthy person, it might spike at 140 mmol/L. In a person with metabolic syndrome or pre-diabetes, the level may go as high as 180 mmol/L. People with diabetes might see it go much higher if they aren't being treated.

You can do a simple test at home with a blood sugar meter and some orange juice, to see how your body responds to blood sugar. Drink an 8-ounce glass of orange juice and wait two hours. Then check your blood sugar and see how high it rises. If it's higher than 140 mmol/L, then you definitely have issues with blood sugar. But again – you probably don't want it going to 140 in the first place.

Fluctuating blood sugar levels will cause fluctuating levels of stress hormones as well. This is independent of other methods used to control stress like medication. We can avoid this problem by following a keto diet. The keto diet will keep blood sugar levels confined to a narrow range. As a result, stress hormones released in response to fluctuating blood sugars will also be consistent as well, reducing overall stress on the body and keeping you healthier.

Even those with high fasting blood sugars will find that they don't experience any spikes on keto, and even before their fasting blood sugar levels improve they will see better A1C values. For example, if you are pre-diabetic and typically have a fasting blood sugar of 120, you will probably find that eating keto meals your blood sugar only bounces around between 120 and 130, rather than dropping to 100 and then spiking to 180 like it would when eating a carbohydrate-rich diet.

Try doing a second test to see how your body responds with a high fat meal. Before eating, take your blood sugar to get a baseline number. Then eat a fatty meal, with macros of fat, protein, and carbohydrates in proper proportion. Then two hours after taking your first bite retake your blood sugar and check the results. You will find that it will be very close to your baseline number, in contrast to the results you're going to see when doing the orange juice test.

Chapter 12: Keto and Intermittent Fasting

Many people like to incorporate fasting into their keto lifestyle. This can be beneficial for increasing weight loss, and we will see why in a minute. However, it's important to note that fasting is not required for a keto lifestyle. The contents of this chapter are entirely optional.

Fasting Overview

Fasting has been used since the beginning of time as a means of attaining optimal health. Surprisingly, the body may be adapted to some level of fasting. During prehistoric times, game animals and fruits and vegetables were in short supply at times. If human beings were so fragile that they required constant food consumption, they would have vanished a long time ago, and we wouldn't be here today having this conversation. If it took a few extra days to hunt down an animal to get valuable fats and proteins, then the body had to be adapted to being able to go for short periods without food.

It turns out that fasting can be good for you. As always, you should check with your doctor first before starting a fasting program. In the keto world, we call this intermittent fasting because it's something you'll do periodically but not all the time. The benefits that have been tied to fasting are numerous and include:

- Increased weight loss
- Stabilized blood sugars
- Lower blood pressure
- Longer lifespan

- Reduction and even reversal of type 2 diabetes

Diabetics, in particular, should speak to their doctor before adopting a fasting program. Intermittent fasting can have important implications for medications used to treat diabetes. Intermittent fasting also shouldn't be used if you're underweight or have other serious problems such as cancer.

However, if you're in the proper health to incorporate fasting, it's something that you'll want to consider adding to your keto lifestyle.

How Keto Can Be Correlated with Fasting

It's when we look into the details of fasting that we find its connection to the keto diet. You probably won't be surprised. After all, what happens when your body isn't getting a lot of carbohydrates that it can use for energy? Your body makes ketones. So, what happens when we're fasting, and not taking in any carbohydrates?

You guessed it – when you're fasting your body makes ketones to keep energy levels up. Fasting also works as the early stages of keto when you're not used to it. If you've been eating a high carbohydrate diet, fasting will leave you feeling low on energy and cause brain fog. That's because your body requires time to adjust and make ketones that can be used for energy. If you're already following a ketogenic diet, you aren't going to have near as many problems with this which means that you'll be a lot more comfortable fasting. Your body is already keto-adjusted meaning that you're producing and deriving energy from ketones.

The fact is everyone fasts already! Each day, you go a long time between eating dinner and breakfast. Typically, this period lasts from 8-12 hours or even longer. The word breakfast literally means *breakfast*.

The principles behind intermittent fasting are quite simple. Your body stores excess calories as body fat. It does this because, in the long eons of history that preceded us, people who could call on stored energy to stay alive during periods of food deprivation are the ones who had offspring and passed on their genes. If you couldn't gather energy from stored body fat, you'd be in major trouble if the hunting team couldn't find a deer on a given day.

When you fast, all that happens is your body draws on the reserves of stored fats to produce the energy it needs. Here you can see why those who aren't keto-adapted will find fasting more challenging to deal with. Their bodies aren't used to using ketones to burn energy, and so fasting can make them feel tired, weak, irritable, and bring on brain fog. The bottom line is they get keto flu when they fast.

However, if you've already been doing keto, then your body is already making ketones. It's going to find that using your body fat to get energy is an easy transition.

Having some body fat is normal. A person with zero body fat would be a strange sight indeed, and if they tried fasting, they'd end up burning whatever muscle they had. This is an extreme example but it's one reason that underweight people shouldn't take up fasting. The bottom line is that having some body fat is normal and healthy.

How is body fat created? The body has a natural process that converts excess calories into fat that can be utilized for energy later. It's not all that different than someone who is financially literate and saves for a rainy day.

Let's think about how the financially prepared person conducts their lives. Suppose for simplicity that Sally earns $100 a month. The person who is careful with their finances realizes that they may not always make $100 a month. They may lose their job, come down with a serious illness, or there may be an economic crisis. They also recognize that in old age if they want to maintain the kind of lifestyle they're used to, they'll need to save money for retirement.

So, Sally plans her life into such a way that she only spends $80 a month on living expenses and entertainment. Each month she puts the excess $20 into her piggy bank. After doing this for three years or 36 months, she has $720 in her piggy bank. This is a stored reserve she can call upon in emergencies, or to use when she retires.

Now consider lazy Joe. He has a job that pays $100 a month too, but he blows all his money. Each month he saves nothing or very little, going out to eat and buying fancy cars. Now and then he puts a few cents in his piggy bank. After three years, he's only got $75 in his bank account.

Then an economic recession hits and both Sally and Joe lose their jobs. Joe is a nervous wreck. He realizes that if he doesn't get a new job fast, he's in big trouble. He starts making plans to sell all his cars, but he can't find buyers because everyone else is hurting too. In a few weeks Joe runs through his $75 and is at the employment office filing for the $10 a month unemployment benefit. Joe, is going to have to curtail his lifestyle in order to survive severely.

Sally, on the other hand, can comfortably spend her money at the same level for several months without worry. She simply looks for a new job and rides out the crisis, living off the funds stored in her piggy bank.

The body is quite similar to this situation. Your body stores fat away when you consume excess calories each day. Of course, unlike finances, some body fat is a good thing but too much causes trouble.

Joe, on the other hand, is like someone who's underweight. They don't have any fat reserves, and so fasting isn't a good deal for them. Joe had to go on unemployment to get *some* money. Like Joe, an underweight person will start burning muscle mass to get some energy. Basically, they will waste away their body.

So how does it actually work?

When you eat food, your body releases insulin along with digestive enzymes. Insulin helps the body take up blood sugar and also acts to help store body fat. There are two major effects:

- Insulin causes sugar to be stored in the liver. It's stored as glycogen and can be released during times of starvation to keep blood sugar levels up. Since glycogen is bound to 3 or 4 water molecules, storing sugar in the liver causes you to put on "water weight."

- Insulin also causes the liver to make fat. The reason is that they livers ability to store glycogen is limited. It can also save some fat, and it can also make fat and then release it into the bloodstream. This latter process is how we get fat.

By now you recognize how everything in the keto puzzle fits together. If you're on keto, you're going to have lower insulin levels, and so your liver will be making less fat.

Remember that the liver has a limited capacity to store glycogen. But we all know that our bodies have an unlimited ability (well virtually unlimited) to store body fat. So, when you're consuming excess calories and your glycogen stores are filled, your body puts the rest away in body fat.

Now that we understand how the body creates and stores fat when excess calories are consumed, let's take a look at what happens when the reverse happens. That is supposed we don't consume any calories at all.

If you're not eating at all, your insulin levels are going to drop. In addition, your blood glucose levels will drop. Your body will then try to find ways to keep your energy levels up, and the first place it's going to look is for glucose. If you're not eating there aren't any outside sources, so your body begins to pull out glycogen, the starches store in your liver (and in muscle cells).

Glycogen can be broken down to make blood sugar and provide energy for the body. Of course, there is a limited supply, so this process only works for a short period. You can exercise too and cut that period way down by burning off all the sugar.

Glycogen stores can power the body for about a day, maybe a day and a half. After that, your body has to call on stored body fat. Most people don't go without food long enough for this process to play out. If you go a few hours without eating, but then replenish your food stores, then you're never going to be in the energy saving mode. At best you'll burn some of the glycogen you have stored.

Intermittent fasting is a way for you to enter the "starvation" state and start burning fat for fuel – your body fat. There are several different methods that people have developed to implement intermittent fasting.

The first method is called 16/8 fasting. This is a pretty simple rule – you limit your eating to 8 hours per day. Then you fast for 16 hours, only consuming water during that time (certainly no alcohol). Since you're eating every day and just restricting the time you consume food to 8 hours, this is a pretty simple way to add fasting to your lifestyle. It's a recommended way for beginners to incorporate fasting.

For example, you can eat dinner between 7:30 PM and 8:00 PM. Then don't eat again until noon the next day. That will give your body a 16 hour fast.

Some experts advise women to use a shorter fasting window, probably 14-15 hours.

The next type of fasting is called 5:2. This is a more advanced and more difficult way to incorporate fasting into your diet. The 5:2 method involves fasting two days per week. It's not necessary to avoid eating at all; practitioners advise consuming a minimal number of calories on fasting days, usually in the range of 500-600 calories.

On the other five days, you eat normally.

So far there hasn't been any scientific proof to demonstrate that 5:2 fasting is better than 16/8 fasting. Moreover, if you're on a ketogenic diet, the benefits of 5:2 fasting are dubious because you're in ketosis already.

The next method of fasting is popularly known as *eat, stop eat*. This involves a complete 24 hour fast. You can choose when to start your 24-hour fast, but it's recommended that you start after eating dinner one night and then don't eat again for 24 hours. You can do this once or twice a week.

This fits in with keto better than the 5:2 method and seems to be quite effective, but may be too much for a lot of people. During the 24-hour fasting period, you don't consume any food products. Simply drink water. For many people, this type of fasting will require a great deal of discipline.

Alternate day fasting involves fasting one day and then eating the next. Some practitioners of this type of fasting follow the 5:2 plan of eating about 500 calories on fasting days. Of course, if you're consuming food, you're not really fasting.

The *warrior diet* is a variation of the 24-hour fasting plan. Using the warrior diet, you only eat once per day. You're advised to consume a large meal, so that you get all of your calories in one sitting. You probably don't want to do this at breakfast, but can do it at lunch or dinner. It's generally advised that you eat your big meal at dinner so that you're consuming all of your calories before going to sleep for the night, so will save some for the next day. The idea is to put your body in a fasting state so that the excess is burned off during the daytime when you're not eating.

There are many different methods of intermittent fasting, and you might have to experiment to see what works best in your case since we're all different. However, it's important to note that with keto the extreme methods of fasting aren't generally necessary. When you're on keto, you're already burning ketones, and have also already depleted excess glycogen stores.

Possible Benefits from Fasting

Let's begin with the obvious. If you engage in intermittent fasting, you're consuming fewer calories. So, you'll experience some level of weight loss. You can accelerate your keto diet plan by adding some intermittent fasting.

It's long been believed that fasting was a way to 'detoxify' the body. That perception is largely correct. Even if you're not eliminating specific 'toxins,' fasting helps detoxify the body in subtle but important ways.

One of the most important ways is that it helps you maintain lower and more stable blood sugar levels. Your insulin level is also reduced. So, in a sense, you're detoxifying your body from its toxins. Insulin isn't really a toxin, but too much of it has toxic effects on the body.

If done properly, intermittent fasting will help you specifically lost body fat. You shouldn't go right into intermittent fasting if you're a keto beginner, as you can lower your glycogen stores simply by adopting a keto diet. Then you'll be able to use intermittent fasting to accelerate the loss of excess body fat.

If you want to do one of the more extreme fasting methods, you can gradually ease into it. Consider starting with the 16/8 method. This is something that most people will be pretty comfortable doing, especially after they're in ketosis. Then one day per week, you can gradually expand the time fasting. The first time you might go 17/7, and then work up to 16/6. The goal is to reach a full 24 hour fast once per week eventually. After you've done that you can add a second day of 24-hour fasting if desired.

While you need to check with your doctor first, doing intermittent fasting can have dramatic effects on those who have type 2 diabetes. Fasting can have major impacts that stabilize blood sugar levels and reduce your blood sugar. Some people even claim to cure their diabetes using intermittent fasting in combination with a ketogenic diet.

Some other benefits that people have associated with intermittent fasting include:

- Weight loss
- Lower blood sugar and cholesterol
- Lower insulin levels
- Burning fat and not muscle
- Increased mental clarity (probably comes from utilizing ketones)
- Increased growth hormones
- Reduced triglycerides

Another possible benefit is the so-called Autophagy. This is a cellular process that involves what might be described as a home cleaning. Your body's immune machinery will go through the body and clear out all the old dysfunctional cells. It is believed that intermittent fasting may trigger or increase this process, helping you achieve a healthier state.

Determining If Fasting Is for You

It's important to note that fasting is not for everyone. It takes discipline and at first, it's going to make you feel tired, irritable and uncomfortable. We will note however that if you're already doing the keto diet, the negative consequences of fasting will be minimized if you experience them at all.

First, let's review who should not be fasting. Frankly, the list of people who should not be fasting include:

- Type 1 diabetics
- Type 2 diabetics on insulin or drugs like metformin that manage blood sugar levels
- Underweight people
- People with serious illnesses like cancer

Well, we've been a little to absolutist. It's possible for type 2 diabetics to engage in fasting, but you should talk about it with your doctor first and adjust your medications and dosing schedule as necessary. The same advice applies to those with cancer, although recent research has rediscovered the fact that cancer cells feed on sugar, so depriving your cancer cells might assist in your treatment plan. Again, talk to your doctor if this describes your situation.

Beyond a few specific subgroups of people, determining if fasting for you is a matter of taste. It's important to note that you don't need to fast to get results from a ketogenic diet, but fasting may speed the results you're looking for and help you maintain a healthier lifestyle.

If you're unsure about fasting but are interested in it, the best thing to do is try to work it in gradually and see how your body reacts. As noted in the previous section, you can slowly ease your way into a 24 hour fast. Alternatively, simply to 16/8 fasting. This method of fasting –when done in conjunction with a keto diet – is pretty gentle. If you do not have diabetes on insulin, you can do 16/8 fasting without giving it any thought. You probably won't even know you're fasting once you've been on the keto diet for any length of time.

Thinking about ketosis, you can see why 16/8 fasting would give a person eating a "normal" diet the blues. When you're eating a diet with a large amount of carbohydrates and not on ketosis, you need to feed yourself sugar to keep going continually. People eating carbs get hungry and they have to eat more often. If you're doing keto one of the first things you might notice is that you're not having hunger pains anymore.

But if you're still eating "normally," your body continually experiences blood sugar peaks and crashes. Through the night your blood sugar gradually drops (unless your pre-diabetic or diabetic, but remember they have trouble using their blood sugar for energy). So, in the morning people are often famished and need to eat and get their blood sugar back up. Far too many people make things even worse by consuming sweets with breakfast, eating sugar-laden donuts or breakfast cereals. And remember even so-called "whole grains" are nothing but sugar, it's just packaged in such a way that it's a little bit harder to get to so takes longer to digest. Whole grains might result in blood sugar spikes that come on more gradually and last longer – but they still create a rise in blood sugar. That simple fact can't be avoided.

Keep in mind that fasting means fasting. You don't want to ruin it by consuming any calories. If you find you need to drink coffee while fasting, you'll have to do it without cream and sweetener (and never sugar –fasting or not). It's best to stick to water while fasting.

If getting up in the morning and going without your coffee and cream is too much to bear, consider doing a 16/8 plan where your 8 hours of eating begins at 8 or 9 in the morning. Just remember that you'll have to schedule your last meal accordingly. If you start consuming at 9 AM, you'll have to be done eating by 5 PM.

Many will find that an occasional 24 hour fast works better for them. You can limit this to one day per week if you find that the impact is too stressful. In any case, plan ahead and test and retest.

- First, get yourself adjusted to keto. Don't start fasting until you're in ketosis and have gotten over the "keto flu" if it's impacting you.

- Try the 16/8 fasting plan first. It's very easy to implement. But remember if you wait until noon to eat your first meal but have morning coffee with cream, you're not fasting. Fasting means not consuming any calories.

- Experiment with different methods. Some people will benefit from or tolerate different ways of fasting.

- The advantage of a once or twice a week fast, or a 5:2 style of fasting, is that you're not fasting all the time.

- If fasting isn't really your thing, but you'd like to enjoy the benefits, try occasionally fasting. Maybe you only fast for 24 hours once or twice a month. It's not necessary to fast all the time to get the benefits.

Chapter 13: The Keto Breakfast

Keto means a lot of cooking. But my meal plan and shopping list will make this the most fun part of the diet. Cooking healthy meals that taste good and are wholly satisfying not only feeds the body, it feeds the soul. Treat yourself and sit down to well-prepared keto meals made with the highest quality ingredients you can afford. It makes a difference, I assure you.

What follows is a 7-day plan. Your first week of keto dieting already planned so you can effortlessly transition without the stress of thinking of *what to cook next*. I have even included a list that will take the guesswork out of grocery shopping. Use the weekend to prep as many ingredients as possible. Wash, chop and store vegetables. Cook and divide meat into servings ready to go. Boil all the eggs at once. Gather spill-proof containers to bring all your keto yumminess to the workplace.

Once you get the hang of cooking and eating keto, you'll be able to mix the recipes around and add a few of your own. The key to healthy eating is variety, which is as we all know, is the spice of life.

In this chapter, we'll cover a seven-day breakfast plan with recipes.

Monday
Breakfast: Simple scrambled eggs with tomato slices

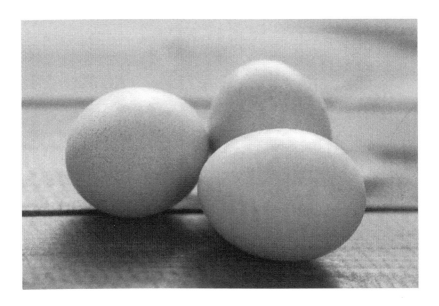

This recipe combines high-quality protein with a low carb tomato to keep you fuller longer.

Variation tip: Substitute your favorite low carb vegetable like spinach or avocado.

Prep Time: 5 minutes
Cook Time: 5 minutes
Servings: 1

What's in it
- Butter (1 ounce)
- Eggs (2)
- Water (1 T)
- Salt and pepper (to taste)
- Small whole tomato (1 qty)

How it's made
- Heat the butter over medium heat in a 10-inch non-stick skillet.
- Crack the eggs into a bowl, add water and beat lightly with a whisk.
- Add the eggs to the skillet and stir until just firm. Be careful not to overcook.
- Slice tomato and serve with the eggs.
- Season with salt and pepper.

Net carbs: 5 grams
Fat: 15 grams
Protein: 11 grams
Sugars: 2.6 grams

Tuesday
Breakfast: Avocado salmon boats

This wholesome breakfast requires no cooking at all, but it's delicious and packed with protein and good fats.

Variation tip: try sour cream instead of mayo.

Prep Time: 5 minutes
Cook Time: None
Servings: 2

What's in it
- Avocados (2 qty)
- Wild caught smoked salmon (6 ounces)
- Mayonnaise (4 T)
- Salt and pepper (to taste)
- Lemon (1 qty)

How it's made
- Carefully cut avocadoes in half. Remove pits.
- Add a tablespoon of sour cream or mayonnaise in the hollow of each avocado half.
- Top each half with equal amounts of salmon
- Sprinkle with salt and pepper
- Cut the lemon into quarters and squeeze over each boat before serving.

Net carbs: 1 gram
Fat: 71 grams
Protein: 16 grams
Sugars: 1 gram

Wednesday

Breakfast: Simple Egg Salad

Egg butter is a savory, flavorful way to start your day.

Variation tip: mix in a little fresh dill or chives.

Prep Time: 5 minutes
Cook Time: 10 minutes
Serves 2

What's in it

- Eggs (4 qty)
- Butter (5 ounces)
- Kosher salt (.5 tsp.)
- Fresh ground pepper (.25 t)

How it's made

- Place eggs in a large pot and fill to cover with cold, filtered water.

- Bring to a rolling boil and let cook for 8-minutes.
- Carefully drain eggs and plunge into a bowl of ice water to stop the eggs from overcooking.
- After the eggs have cooled, peel and chop.
- Combine with butter, kosher salt and fresh ground pepper
- Goes great with lettuce leaves. Also try with avocado slices, smoked salmon, turkey, or ham.

Net carbs: 1 gram
Fat: 69 grams
Protein: 12 grams
Sugars: None

Thursday
Breakfast: Pancakes, The Keto Way

What a treat! Pancakes on the keto diet. If you thought you would miss fluffy pancakes, then try these. They're delicious.

Variation tip: serve with berries and homemade whipped cream, peanut butter or even crumpled, crispy bacon.

Prep Time: 5 minutes
Cook Time: 10 minutes
Serves 4

What's in it
- Eggs (4 qty)
- Cottage cheese (7 ounces)
- Ground psyllium husk powder (At healthy grocery stores 1T)

- Butter (2 ounces)

How it's made

- Mix eggs, cheese and psyllium husk powder together and set aside. The mixture will thicken.
- Over medium heat, melt butter in a nonstick skillet. When melted and slightly bubbly, pour 3 T of pancake batter and cook for 4 minutes. Flip and cook for 3 more minutes. Proceed with the rest of the batter.

Net carbs: 5 grams
Fat: 39 grams
Protein: 13 grams
Sugars: 2 grams

Friday
Breakfast: Break the Fast Burrito Bowl

Skip the carbs from the tortilla by putting leftover seasoned beef and veggies into a bowl. So easy.

Variation tip: try different toppings, like salsa.

Prep Time: 5 minutes
Cook Time: 15 minutes
Serves 2

What's in it
- Seasoned ground beef – can use Keto Taco recipe (.5 pounds)
- Prepared riced cauliflower (2 cups)
- Chopped cilantro (2 T)
- Butter (2 t, divided)

- Eggs (3 qty)
- Salt (to taste)
- Pepper (to taste)

How it's made
- Brown and season the beef in a large skillet with a teaspoon of the butter. When done, push to one side.
- Add diced cauliflower and chopped cilantro. Season with salt. Push to the side.
- Melt a teaspoon of butter in the open space of the skillet.
- Beat the eggs and add to the butter. Scramble in the skillet. If your skillet isn't large enough for this step, use a separate pan.
- Mix everything together. Taste.
- Season with salt and pepper if necessary.

Net carbs: 4 grams
Fat: 14 grams
Protein: 34 grams
Sugars: 2 grams

Saturday
Breakfast: Jalapeno Bacon Egg Cups

Have a little extra time this morning for some self-care? Try my Jalapeno Bacon Egg Cups. These spicy cups will wake your senses and send you out the door with a spring in your step.

Variation tip: replace jalapenos with green onions.

Prep Time: 5 minutes
Cook Time: 20 minutes
Serves 4

What's in it
- Nitrate-free bacon, cooked and crumbled (5 ounces)
- Eggs (12 qty)
- Cheddar, shredded (6 ounces)
- Jalapeno (2 qty)
- Salt (to taste)
- Pepper (to taste)

How it's made
- Turn the oven on so that it preheats to 350 degrees F.
- Cut jalapeno in half, lengthwise, and remove seeds. Chop 1 jalapeno and slice the other.
- Beat eggs with a whisk and add cheese
- Grease a muffin tin with fat of choice and layer the bottom with the chopped jalapeno and bacon. Pour the egg mixture into each muffin well.
- Each muffin gets a slice of the other jalapeno on top.
- Pop into the hot oven for about 20 minutes. Eggs should no longer look wet. When done, remove from oven and let cool.
- Serve

Net carbs: 3 grams
Fat: 39 grams
Protein: 35 grams
Sugars: 0 grams

Sunday
Breakfast: Classic bacon and eggs for one

What's it in it (for one):
- 2 eggs
- 1¼ oz. bacon, in slices
- cherry tomatoes (optional)
- fresh parsley (optional)

How it's made:
- Fry bacon in a pan on medium-high heat. Remove and set aside, leaving bacon fat in the pan.
- Crack eggs and place in pan, cooking and seasoning to taste. You can cook them scrambled, sunny side up or any way you like. Optionally you can add a small bit of cream to up the fat content of your meal and add extra flavor.
- Slice cherry tomatoes in half, and optionally quickly fry in the bacon grease.

- Put the entire contents of the pan onto your serving plate. Optionally, substitute two strawberries or blackberries for the cherry tomatoes.

Net carbs: 1 gram
Fat: 22 grams
Protein: 15 grams
Sugars: 0 grams but depends on optional fruits or vegetables

Chapter 14: The Keto Lunch

In this chapter, we'll provide a seven-day menu that you can use for some easy to make but extremely delicious keto lunches.

Monday
Lunch: Keto Meatballs

Make these ahead of time because these delicious meatballs are freezable. Take a few to work along with some sugar-free marinara sauce and zoodles (zucchini noodles) for a delicious keto lunch.

Variation tip: change the seasonings to make different flavors, like taco or barbecue.

Prep Time: 5 minutes
Cook Time: 18 minutes

Servings: 4
What's in it

- Grass-fed ground beef (1 pound)
- Chopped fresh parsley (1.5 t)
- Onion powder (.75 t)
- Garlic powder (.75 t)
- Kosher salt (.75 t)
- Fresh ground black pepper (.5 t)

How it's made

- Turn oven to 400-degrees F to preheat.
- Using parchment paper, line a baking sheet.
- Put beef into a medium-sized glass bowl with other ingredients and mix with hands until just combined. Avoid over-mixing as this will result in tough meatballs.
- Roll into 8 meatballs and place on the lined baking sheet.
- Bake for 15-18 minutes until done all the way through.

Net carbs: 3 grams
Fat: 17 grams
Protein: 11 grams
Sugars: 2 grams

Tuesday

Lunch: Mason Jar Salad

So colorful and full of flavor. This salad is portable. Use any vegetable you have on hand.

Variation tip: try different kinds of protein, cheese or seeds.

Prep Time: 10 minutes
Cook Time: None
Servings: 1

What's in it
- Cooked, diced chicken (4 ounces)
- Baby spinach (1/6 ounce)
- Cherry tomatoes (1/6 ounce)
- Bell pepper (1/6 ounce)
- Cucumber (1/6 ounce)

- Green onion (1/2 qty)
- Extra virgin olive oil (4 T)

How it's made
- Chop vegetables.
- Stuff spinach at the bottom of jar.
- Layer the rest of the vegetables.
- Keep olive oil in a separate container until ready to eat.

Net carbs: 4 grams
Fat: 55 grams
Protein: 71 grams
Sugars: 1 gram

Wednesday
Lunch: The Smoked Salmon Special

This may be the easiest lunch special ever. Flavorful, smoky, pink salmon poses on your plate next to dark, green spinach as a feast for the eyes and the body.

Variation tip: serve with arugula or cabbage.

Prep Time: 5 minutes
Cook Time: None
Serves 2

What's in it
- Wild caught smoked salmon (.5 ounces)
- Mayonnaise (generous dollop)
- Baby spinach (large handful)
- Extra virgin olive oil (.5 T)

- Lime wedge (1 qty)
- Kosher salt (to taste)
- Fresh ground pepper (to taste)

How it's made
- Place salmon (or any fatty fish like sardines or mackerel) and spinach on a plate.
- Add a large spoonful of mayonnaise and the lime wedge.
- Drizzle oil atop the baby spinach (or try arugula or cabbage shredded as if for slaw)
- Sprinkle with a little salt and pepper.

Net carbs: None
Fat: 109 grams
Protein: 105 grams
Sugars: None

Thursday

Lunch: Ham and Brie Plate

Like a hoagie, but way better.

Variation tip: this is a mix-and-match situation, so experiment with different cheeses and cold cuts.

Prep Time: 5 minutes
Cook Time: None
Serves 2

What's in it
- Ham, sliced thin (9 ounces)
- Brie cheese (5 ounces)
- Anchovies (2/3 ounces
- Green pesto (2 T)
- Kalamata olives (10 qty)

- Baby spinach (1/6 ounce)
- Mayonnaise (.5 cup)
- Fresh basil leaves (10 qty)

How it's made
- Place ingredients on a plate with a serving of mayonnaise.

Net carbs: 6 grams
Fat: 103 grams
Protein: 40 grams
Sugars: 0 grams

Friday
Lunch: Creamy Avocado and Bacon with Goat Cheese Salad

Salad gets an upgrade when crave-able avocado and goat cheese are combined with crispy bacon and crunchy nuts. Fast and good for lunch or dinner.

Variation tip: use different fresh herbs in the dressing.

Prep Time: 10 minutes
Cook Time: 20 minutes
Serves 4

What's in it
Salad:
- Goat cheese (1 8-ounce log)
- Bacon (.5 pound)
- Avocados (2 qty)

- Toasted walnuts or pecans (.5 cup)
- Arugula or baby spinach (4 ounces)

Dressing:
- One-half lemon, juiced
- Mayonnaise (.5 cup)
- Extra virgin olive oil (.5 cup)
- Heavy whipping cream (2 T)
- Kosher salt (to taste)
- Fresh ground pepper (to taste)

How it's made
- Line a baking dish with parchment paper.
- Preheat oven to 400 degrees F.
- Slice goat cheese into half-inch rounds and put in baking dish. Place on an upper rack in preheated oven until golden brown.
- Cook bacon until crisp. Chop into pieces
- Slice avocado and place on greens. Top with bacon pieces and add goat cheese rounds.
- Chop nuts and sprinkle on the salad.
- For dressing, combine lemon juice, mayo, extra virgin olive oil and whipping cream. Blend with countertop or immersion blender.
- Season to taste with kosher salt and fresh ground pepper.

Net carbs: 6 grams
Fat: 123 grams
Protein: 27 grams
Sugars: 1 gram

Saturday
Lunch: Chicken Noodle-less Soup

All the comfort of a classic soup without the carbs. How comforting.

Variation tip: use the meat from a rotisserie chicken.

Prep Time: 10 minutes
Cook Time: 20 minutes
Serves 4

What's in it
- Butter (.25 cup)
- Celery (1 stalk)
- Mushrooms (3 ounces)
- Garlic, minced (1 clove)

- Dried minced onion (1 T)
- Dried parsley (1 t)
- Chicken stock (4 cups)
- Kosher salt (.5 t)
- Fresh ground pepper (.25 t)
- Carrot, chopped (1 qty)
- Chicken, cooked and diced (2.5 cups or 1.5 pounds of chicken breast)
- Cabbage, sliced (1 cups)

How it's made
- Put large soup pot on medium heat and melt butter.
- Slice the celery and mushrooms and add, along with dried onion to the pot.
- Add parsley, broth, carrot, kosher salt and fresh pepper. Stir.
- Simmer until veggies are tender.
- Stir in cooked chicken and sliced cabbage. Simmer until cabbage is tender, about 8 to 12 minutes.

Net carbs: 4 grams
Fat. 40 grams
Protein: 33 grams
Sugars: 1 gram

Sunday
Lunch: Cheese and turkey rollups

What's in it:
- 3 slices of turkey lunchmeat
- 3 slices of cheese (your choice)
- ½ avocado
- 3 slices of cucumber
- a quarter cup of blueberries
- handful of almonds

How it's made:

- Using your cheese as bread, make "turkey rolls" by rolling up the turkey meat, a few slices of avocado, and the cucumber slices.
- Enjoy, and snack on the blueberries and almonds.

Contains 13 net carbs.

Chapter 15: Keto at Dinner

Monday

Dinner: Beef short ribs in a slow cooker

With a little prep, you will have a hot meal waiting for you at the end of a long day.

Variation tip: serve over diced cauliflower or with celery.

Prep Time: 15 minutes
Cook Time: 4 hours
Servings: 4

What's in it

- Boneless short ribs or bone-in (2 pounds)
- Kosher salt (to taste)
- Fresh ground pepper (to taste)

- Extra virgin olive oil (2 T)
- Chopped white onion (1 qty)
- Garlic (3 cloves)
- Bone broth (1 cup)
- Coconut aminos (2 T)
- Tomato paste (2 T)
- Red wine (1.5 cups)

How it's made
- In a large skillet over medium heat, add olive oil. Season meat with salt and pepper. Brown both sides.
- Add broth and browned ribs to slow cooker
- Put remaining ingredients into the skillet.
- Bring to a boil and cook until onions are tender. About 5 minutes.
- Pour over ribs.
- Set to 4 to 6 hours on high or 8 to 10 hours on low.

Net carbs: 1 gram
Fat: 63 grams
Protein: 24 grams
Sugars: 1 gram

Tuesday
Dinner: Chicken Thighs with Garlic and Parmesan Cheese

Tastes like chicken wings but heartier.

Variation tip: try cooking in a cast iron skillet for superb searing. Dried basil instead of Italian seasoning would work nicely.

Prep Time: 5 minutes
Cook Time: 35 minutes
Serves 4

What's in it
- Bone in chicken thighs (6 qty)
- Italian seasoning (1 T)
- Shredded parmesan cheese (1 T)
- Garlic cloves, chopped (1 qty)
- Kosher salt (to taste)
- Fresh ground pepper (to taste)

How it's made
- Turn oven to 450 degrees F to preheat
- Pull the skin away from the top of the thigh to create a pocket.
- Mix together Italian seasoning, shredded parmesan cheese, garlic, 1/8 teaspoon of kosher salt, fresh ground pepper and scant drops of extra virgin olive oil.
- Divide the mixture between the thighs. Rub evenly under the skin.
- In an ovenproof skillet, heat extra virgin olive oil over medium-high heat.
- Put thighs skin side down and allow to cook for about 5 minutes. Flip and cook for 8 to 10 minutes.
- Transfer the skillet to the hot oven for 15-20 minutes until cooked all the way through.
- Let rest, then serve.

Net carbs: 0.6 grams
Fat: 29 grams
Protein: 27 grams
Sugars: 0 grams

Wednesday
Dinner: Keto Tacos

Tacos get a makeover too. Instead of tortillas, filling is stuffed into zucchini boats. Make extra seasoning to always have on hand for taco meat anytime.

Variation tips: Try different types of cheeses. Serve with salsa.

Prep Time: 15 minutes
Cook Time: 30 minutes
Serves 4

What's in it
- Zucchini (2 qty)
- Extra virgin olive oil (3 T, divided)
- Grass fed ground beef or pork (1 pound)

- Kosher salt (1 t)
- White onion, chopped (.25 cup)
- Chili powder (1 t)
- Cumin (.5 t)
- Oregano (.5 t)
- Shredded cheddar cheese (1.25 cups)

How it's made
- Turn oven to 400 degrees F to preheat.
- Slice zucchini in half lengthwise and scoop out seeds to make boats. Sprinkle with kosher salt. Let sit for about 10 minutes.
- Heat 2 T of extra virgin olive oil in skillet and brown meat.
- Add chili powder, cumin, oregano and salt. Cook until liquid is mostly gone.
- Blot zucchini with a paper towel and put on a baking sheet that has been greased.
- Mix 1/3 of cheese in the seasoned beef.
- Stuff the cheesy beef into the zucchini boats evenly and place in hot oven for about 20 minutes until cheese starts to turn brown. Remove from the oven and let cool for a few minutes.

Net carbs: 6 grams
Fat: 49 grams
Protein: 33 grams
Sugars: 2 grams

Thursday

Dinner: On the go chicken wings with green beans

We decided to incorporate a meal idea here to illustrate how you can build your keto meals when you're pressed for time.

What's In it:
- Pecan smoked chicken wings (frozen, available at WalMart)
- Marketside French Green beans (fresh and packaged for microwaving, available at Walmart.

How it's made:
- Preheat oven to 425.
- Bake chicken wings for 30-35 minutes.
- When chicken wings are almost done, place beans inside a microwave in the bag and cook for 2-3 minutes.

- Take beans out and season with butter or olive oil, and salt and pepper.
- Enjoy with your chicken wings!

Net carbs: 7 grams
Fat: 14 grams per 4 ounces serving of chicken, be sure to add butter or olive oil used
Protein: 14 grams per 4 ounces serving of chicken
Sugars: 3 grams

Friday
Dinner: Minute Steak with Mushrooms and Herb Butter

This dinner comes together fast. Perfect for busy weeknights.

Variation tip: try over any of your favorite vegetables.

Prep Time: 10 minutes
Cook Time: 20 minutes
Serves 4

What's in it
For steaks:
- Minute steaks (8 qty)
- Toothpicks (8 qty)
- Gruyere cheese, cut into sticks (3 ounces)
- Kosher salt (to taste)
- Fresh ground pepper (to taste)

- Butter (2 T)
- Leeks (2 qty)
- Mushrooms (15 ounces)
- Extra virgin olive oil (2 T)

For herb butter:
- Butter (5 ounces)
- Minced garlic cloves (1 qty)
- Garlic powder (.5 T)
- Chopped parsley (4 T)
- Lemon juice (1 t)
- Kosher salt (.5 t)

How it's made
- Combine all herb butter ingredients in a glass bowl. Set aside for at least 15 minutes.
- Slice leeks and mushrooms. Sauté in extra virgin olive oil until lightly brown. Season with salt and pepper. Remove from skillet and keep warm.
- Season steaks with salt and pepper. Place a stick of cheese in the center and roll up steaks, securing with a toothpick.
- Sauté on medium heat for 10 to 15 minutes.
- Pour pan juices on vegetables.
- Plate steaks and vegetables and serve with herb butter.

Net carbs: 6 grams
Fat: 89 grams
Protein: 52 grams
Sugars: 2 grams

Saturday
Dinner: "Breaded" Pork Chops

With crispy, keto friendly breading, this is sure to be a family favorite.

Variation tip: if you can spare the calories, sprinkle with shredded Parmesan cheese.

Prep Time: 5 minutes
Cook Time: 30 minutes
Serves 4

What's in it

- Boneless thin pork chops (4 qty)
- Psyllium husk powder (1 T)
- Kosher salt (.5 t)

- Paprika (.25 t)
- Garlic powder (.25 t)
- Onion powder (.25 t)
- Oregano (.25 t)

How it's made

- Preheat oven to 350 degrees F.
- Dry pork chops with a paper towel.
- Combine the rest of the ingredients in a ziplock bag.
- One at a time, seal the pork chops in the bag and shake to coat.
- Put a wire rack on a baking sheet. Place pork chops on rack.
- Bake in oven for approximately 30 minutes. The thermometer should read 145 degrees F.
- Serve with vegetables or a green salad.

Net carbs: 0 grams
Fat: 9 grams
Protein: 28 grams
Sugars: 0 grams

Sunday
Dinner: Lamb Chops

Celebrate Saturday night with juicy lamb chops served with herbal butter. Perfection.

Variation tip: serve with a simple green salad or other vegetable. Can also substitute pork chops.

Prep Time: 15 minutes
Cook Time: 10 minutes
Serves 4

What's in it

- Lamb chops (8 qty)
- Butter (1 T)
- Extra virgin olive oil (1 T)
- Kosher salt (to taste)
- Fresh ground pepper (to taste)
- Lemon, cut into wedges (1 qty)
- Set chops out to bring to room temperature.
- Sprinkle with kosher salt and fresh ground pepper.
- Heat butter and oil in skillet. Add chops and brown on both sides, 3 to 4 minutes each side.
- Serve with lemon wedges and butter.

Net carbs: 1 gram
Fat: 90 grams
Protein: 44 grams
Sugars: 0 gram

Chapter 16: Eating on the Go

One of the pitfalls facing beginners on the keto diet is eating with other people – this can include eating at home with family members who don't want to join you on keto or going out to eat. We leave it to the reader to work out how they're going to deal with their family members – in this chapter we'll offer some remarks and guidance about eating out.

Managing Keto in Restaurants

There are many distinct issues that you'll be dealing with while eating out. Many of them are so obvious they're not even worth discussing, but for the sake of completeness, we'll mention them. Obviously, you're going to want to avoid eating carbohydrate laden meals. That means to hold the French fries. A medium serving of McDonalds French fries contains 50 grams of carbs. So, eat that and you're done – you've gone way beyond any permissible limits on carbohydrate consumption when it comes to keto. Only 4.6 grams of a medium order of French fries are dietary fiber – so they pack on with net carbs too.

Luckily for us, we not only live in a time when food is convenient and widely available, but we also live in an era when information is king. This will be harder with local restaurants, but large ones and chains have posted complete nutritional information online. Use this information. You can build up a nice detailed list of where you can eat and what you can eat, and how much damage eating a particular place will do to your diet.

Unfortunately, there are not many restaurants that cater to keto, paleo, or low carb eating. So, you're going to have to adapt to them rather than the other way around. One option you can consider if one is located near your office or home is Boston

Market. You'll have to be careful on the side items – but Boston Market offers quarter and half chickens and other meat items like prime rib.

Barbecue places can also be utilized (but more below). You can consume a lot of meat items like chicken, pork ribs, and beef brisket.

One surprising option that might surprise you is fried chicken. Now we offer this with a caveat – we are not suggesting that you should include fried chicken with your keto diet. But if you're in a bind and need some fast food, it might be an option.

For example, according to the Church's Chicken website, they list the following carbohydrate content:

- Leg: 6 carbs
- Wing: 8 carbs
- Thigh: 12 carbs (1 gram of fiber, 11 net carbs)
- Breast: 9 carbs

So, it's possible to eat a meal of fried chicken without completely wrecking your diet. Of course, having more than one piece comes dangerously close – you'll have to watch your vegetable consumption the rest of the day to stay under 30 grams of total carbs.

In hamburger joints, you can always eat the burger without the bun. You can also opt for steak or fish in many restaurants, and only eat vegetables. In Mexican restaurants, if they have it available eat carne asada or carne adovada, which is beef or pork in a spicy sauce that usually has little or no carbohydrates.

In an Indian restaurant, you can opt for kabobs. Note that depending on the local recipe used tandoori chicken might have a lot of carbohydrates. Food items like Chinese are usually entirely out. If you want to eat Chinese, you'll have to consider it on a cheat day.

Sushi can work and can be a healthy option for keto dieters. If you're going to do sushi though you'll need to restrict yourself to *sashimi*, which is plain raw fish. Soy sauce and wasabi are OK to use. Stay away from soups and "salads" that might be enhanced with carbohydrates or sweetened with sugar.

The bottom line is that eating out is very difficult on keto, as the rest of the world hasn't come around to this healthy lifestyle, at least not yet. So, it's probably best to pack a lunch for work or school. If you have to eat out, you might use a keto meter to track directly and see how your body is responding, and what meals cause you to go off ketosis and which ones don't. By process of trial and error you might find some meals that work for you.

Watch Out for Hidden Carbs

If you do find yourself in a position where you have to eat out, one of the biggest dangers is hidden carbs. While everyone else is worrying about butter, they aren't noticing that the chefs are using sugar and starches to "spice up" their food.

Some of these hidden carbs are more obvious than others. The first place where you're going to find hidden carbs is in condiments and sauces. Barbecue sauce as many people know is loaded with sugar. On a teaspoon by teaspoon basis, you're not getting a huge amount of sugar, but if you eat food marinated in different sauces, there is no telling how much you're consuming. On keto, it's important to know how many carbs you're getting.

Another problem is the teriyaki sauce. You can hit a Japanese restaurant and say "hold the rice" but teriyaki sauce has sugar in it, and the amount of sugar will vary. If it's a larger restaurant or chain, you may be able to find out how much sugar is in the sauce, but in most cases it's a guessing game.

Pizza, of course, is completely out. And it's not just the tomato sauce.

Chines food, like Japanese, can be problematic. You might be able to find some dishes that without the rice appear to be meat and vegetables. Two problems come up here – the first is that you're not getting enough fat. What do most Chinese dishes include? Lean meat. Of course, there are oils in the sauces but the second issue is that Chinese sauces usually contain a lot of sugar.

In fact, cooked vegetables in any restaurant can be a problem. Remember restaurants don't care about your health, they only care about creating addicting food that tastes good. So, the "vegetables" might be cooked in a sugar-containing sauce or marinade and it might not be immediately evident that this was done. So, you might be consuming more carbs than you think you are.

Not to be brutal about it, but the bottom line is no matter what eating out can be problematic. It might not be feasible to avoid eating out all the time, but a good rule for a beginner to follow is to use the plan put forward by the Atkins diet. Take at least two weeks (the "induction" phase) where your carbohydrates are severely restricted to twenty grams per day. You can do this for two weeks or up to a month depending on your situation. After that, then you can ease up a bit and start eating out now and then. That way you'll achieve your weight loss goals and not suffer a catastrophic defeat by eating out once in a while.

We've also discussed the possibility of incorporating a "cheat" day here and there. This should also be done after the induction period, but if you include a cheat day, you can schedule it, so it occurs on days you know that you'll be eating out.

Shake and Snack Options

Fortunately, this area of inquiry will be more fruitful than trying to cobble together a low carb meal at a fried chicken outlet. Many viable snack options can fit into a keto diet.

Firstly, consider canned fish. Sardines and mackerel are best for this purpose because they contain high amounts of fat. You can even include something like an avocado with a tin can of fish for a complete lunch. Tuna can be added if the amount of protein in the can is noted as part of your daily intake, and it's consumed with a large amount of fat. You can also get your fat from other sources like cheese, but don't eat the tuna by itself. Anchovies are also good as they are a low calorie but high fat fish, but note the salt content.

Speaking of cheese, it makes a great snack that can be incorporated into a keto diet. There are many kinds of cheese that you can consume including mozzarella cheese sticks, brie, or cheddar. Before consuming cheese be sure to check the nutrition facts to avoid any "hidden" problems. Avoid high protein consumption and any latent carbs.

Next, on the snack list are nuts. This has to be done with care and should be done after an initial "induction" phase in your diet. Macadamia nuts are the preferred choice as they are high fat and low protein. A one-ounce serving is 204 calories with only 2.2 grams of protein. You can consume other kinds of nuts, but you should be aware of the protein and carbs they contain. Nuts are high fiber, so for most varieties net carbs will be low, except for cashews. Try buying snack packs so that you can track the exact number of grams of protein.

Other snacks can be used as well. This includes prosciutto and panino along with deli meats. Keep in mind, however, that your consumption of these foods should be limited. Some contain hidden carbs and, in all cases, you want to track your protein consumption carefully. Eating a high protein meal without accompanying fat will be a problem.

Guacamole is a good snack food to consider, as are avocados in general.

Conclusion

If you're looking for an easy way to lose weight and feel better without having to experience deprivation, the keto diet might be for you. With the keto diet, you can enjoy rich and satisfying foods while still losing weight.

The keto diet is based on a few simple principles. We call the state of burning ketones (fat) for energy ketosis. Getting into ketosis is the first task faced when adopting a keto lifestyle.

First, limit your daily carbohydrate consumption to 20-30 grams per day. Second, define your protein consumption by matching grams consumed to your body mass. The rule to use is to eat at least 0.45 grams of protein per pound of body weight, but don't consume more than 0.5 grams of protein per pound of body weight. It's important not to consume too much protein because then the body will make protein into sugar, raising your blood sugar and defeating ketosis.

After you've planned out your protein and carbohydrates, eat fat. You can eat all the fat you want as long as you're not doing it to excess. But unlike Weight Watchers or other diet plans, you don't need to measure fat or count calories. Simply let your body tell you when you've had enough. If you eat fat until your satiated, then you won't have problems consuming too many calories. If you eat and still feel like you need to eat more – do it. Many beginners on keto get into trouble when they don't eat enough fat.

Keto has many health benefits. These include: losing weight, improved cholesterol, reduced blood sugar, lower triglycerides, and lower insulin levels. Keto can be very helpful for people with pre-diabetes or diabetics, but people on medication should discuss with their doctor first.

Fasting can be incorporated into the keto diet, if it's done correctly. Try out one of the intermittent fasting techniques to help accelerate and maintain weight loss after you're adapted to keto.

Electronic monitors can be very helpful to keep track of your progress at home. If you can afford it, you should get a blood sugar monitor and a ketone monitor. Track your fasting blood sugars and keep track of your ketones, ensuring that they fall within the 1.5-3.0 mmol/dL range. Also, you may want to track your HDL and triglycerides. Home monitors can be used to do this as well, allowing you to monitor progress more frequently and avoid unnecessary trips to the doctor's office.

Lastly, remember to keep a journal. It's important to keep track of your progress and helps you note not only how your triglycerides may be improving, but if you write down what you actually eat and find out you're not losing weight, it will make it easier to pinpoint problem areas where you can improve. One common mistake is people often consume too much protein and don't adjust their protein levels downward when they start losing weight.

Well, that does it for the book. I want to thank you for reading and hope that you found the book informative and that it will help you excel on your keto journey. If you've enjoyed the book, a review on Amazon would be much appreciated!

Bonus: Shopping list ideas

Building up your cabinet to serve keto compliant meals isn't all that difficult, but beginners often have trouble coming up with a complete shopping list. Here are some ideas to help get you started. The ingredients on this list can be used to make the recipes included in this book.

Produce
Baby spinach 1 pound
Cucumber 1
Bell pepper 1
Tomato 5
Cherry tomatoes 1 pint
Cabbage 1 head
White onions 3
Red onion 1
Green onion 1 bunch
Leeks 2 qty
Zucchini 2
Celery 1 stalk
Parsley 1 bunch
Cilantro 1 bunch
Basil 1 bunch
Garlic 2 heads
Avocados 4
Lemons 3
Limes 1
Jalapenos 2
Sliced mushrooms 15 ounces
Broccoli
Cauliflower
Asparagus

Pantry

Extra virgin olive oil
Anchovies
Green pesto
Tomato paste 1 tube
Tomato sauce 7 ounces
Kosher salt
Pepper
Chili powder
Cumin
Onion powder
Garlic powder
Paprika
Italian seasoning
Crushed red pepper flakes
Oregano
Dried minced onions
Dried parsley
Bone broth/stock 5 cups
Mayonnaise
Coconut aminos
Kalamata olives 1 jar
Walnuts or pecans ½ cup
Ground psyllium husk powder
Canned sardines
Canned mackerel (try canned in olive oil, better flavor)
Canned tuna
Coconut oil

Frozen

Riced cauliflower 10 ounces

Chicken wings (opt for low carb varieties, avoid honey barbecue)
Refrigerated/Dairy

Eggs 25 qty
Butter 1.75 pound (if you can, opt for butter from grass-fed cows)
Parmesan cheese, shredded
Ricotta cheese 2/3 cups
Cheddar cheese, shredded 4 cups
Gruyere cheese (3 ounces)
Cottage cheese 7 ounces
Goat cheese 8 ounces
Brie cheese 5 ounces
Heavy whipping cream
Coconut cream

Meat/Butcher

Grass fed ground beef 1.75 pounds
Minute steaks (8 qty)
Boneless or bone-in beef short ribs 2 pounds
Wild caught smoked salmon 12 ounces
Boneless chicken breast 1.75 pounds
Boneless thin pork chops 4 qty
Bone in chicken thighs 6 qty
Lamb chops 8 qty
Chorizo, 1 pound
Bacon 12 ounces
Pork loin
Pork sirloin steaks
Sea bass
Fresh sardines
Sausage (check carb content)
Rib eye steaks

Lamb —leg of lamb, shoulder and leg steaks
Deli and snacks
Ham 9 ounces
Sliced turkey
Prosciutto
Cheese sticks

Beverages
Red wine
White wine
Coffee
Tea
Bottled water
Soda water

Keto Meal Prep:

The everyday quick, cheap, and easy cookbook guide you need! Become a master with these 50 best ketogenic diet recipes and burn fat in just 21 days! (Beginners friendly)

By: Serena Baker

only for informational purposes and should thus be thought of as universal. As befitting its nature, it is presented without assurance regarding its prolonged validity or interim quality. Trademarks that are mentioned are done without written consent and can in no way be considered an endorsement from the trademark holder.

Introduction

Congratulations on buy your copy of the *Keto Meal Prep: The everyday quick, cheap, and easy cookbook guide you need! Become a master with these 50 best ketogenic diet recipes and burn fat in just 21 days!*
I'm delighted that you have chosen to add more recipes to your Keto diet plan.

It is alright if you are just starting with the Keto diet as this cookbook comes with tips for how to begin your new lifestyle and all the basics about the Keto diet. This information will also be helpful reminders to the dedicated Keto dieters, and may give you further information that you can incorporate into your life. The plan goes by many different names such as the low-carb diet, the Keto diet, and the low-carbohydrate diet &high-fat (LCHF) diet plan. But we will keep it simple and call it the Keto diet in this cookbook.

There are tips on what foods you should eat and the ones to avoid as well as ways to store your new Keto recipe meals safely so that you can save time and money. Included as well are the health benefits of following this lifestyle and helpful information for people suffering from specific ailments.

The recipes in this book are easy to follow, and most are made for beginners and can even be made under half an hour, as I know time is essential to every person in this day in age. The meals and snacks inside will add variety to your diet if you have gotten tired of the same old recipes.

Some of the recipes may require a few more steps, but each recipe will provide you with an estimated preparation and cooking time, amount of servings, and a list of nutritional values including calories, net carbohydrates, protein, and fats. It is all laid out for you, in a simple to follow list of instructions to get started on incorporating the Keto diet in your life today.

There are plenty of books on the Keto diet in the market today and thanks again for choosing this one! Every effort was made to ensure that it is full of as much useful information as possible.

Chapter 1: The Basics of the Keto Diet for the Beginner

What is the Keto Diet

The word *Keto* comes from the term *ketogenic* which is a medical expression that defines the state of the body when ketones are produced from fat consumption. Your body ordinarily produces glucose from carbohydrate intake which is where the body gets its source of energy. However, if carb ingestion is too high, it will result in weight gain and health complications.

For example, the standard American diet contains approximately 60% of carbs. Compare this to the Keto diet where you will be consuming about 75% healthy fats and keep carb intake around 5%. When you make this switch in your diet, you will generally see the weight loss benefits due to your body producing the ketones, which is precisely the goal of the Keto diet.

So the simplest way to explain the Keto diet is when you are restricting your carb intake, then your body will enter the state of ketosis, which will make your body into a fat burning machine!

As with any change in lifestyle, consult your doctor about your specific needs, as the Keto diet is not for everyone.

How does the Keto Diet Work

The goal of Keto is to reach the point where your body is creating ketones while you are in ketosis and to stay there. So how does this process work? This explanation will shed some light to understand your first goal during the Keto diet better.

Ketones are an important chemical in the Keto diet, because it is the ultimate goal for your liver to create these ketones, which is the result of fat in your body being recycled for fuel. This process occurs when there is a deficit of insulin in your body. The insulin is responsible for transferring the glucose or sugars into the energy you need every day to function properly.

Most of the information that has been studied about Ketosis is for people who have fasted. This is due to the process of Ketosis starting when the body has expended the carbs present, which in turn makes the liver start creating ketones to make up the deficit. When you fast for longer than 72 hours, the liver will produce even more ketones.

Now, you are not going to be fasting by a long shot. You are going to be transforming your relationship with food so that you can easily reach your goals without feeling hungry. The Keto diet keeps your carb intake low so that it tricks your body that you are essentially fasting, which keeps your liver to produce the ketones needed for your body to stay in Ketosis.

There is a balance with how many macronutrients you consume to keep the level of Ketosis you desire in your body, on the Keto diet. If you, for example, eat too many proteins, your insulin levels will rise. As we learned, this will take your body out of Ketosis. As a result, the insulin will create the sugars that your body is used to using for fuel and stops the production of ketones by the liver.

Who Should Avoid the Keto Diet

Certain individuals should consult their doctor before planning on switching to the Keto diet. Even if you do not have any of these medical issues and you have any doubts, it does not hurt to talk to your doctor. The following are people who are at high risk according to many research studies:

- Individuals who have had gallbladder removal surgery

- A history with any diagnosed eating disorder

- Diagnosed with Multiple Sclerosis

- Thyroid Disease Sufferers

- Patients with kidney damage

- Breastfeeding or Pregnant

- Those with risk or diagnosed with heart disease

For some of these ailments, there is conflicting information, and there has not been conclusive evidence supporting the Keto diet through scientific research. Again, it is best to talk to your doctor if you do suffer from any of these ailments, but you still believe it may be a good change for you.

How to Start

First off, congratulations on making the switch to the Keto diet! It may feel overwhelming at first, but this will give you a simple guide to follow to get started on the Keto diet today. This will also be a helpful tool for the current followers of the Keto diet, as it may have new information that you can incorporate into what you are already exercising in your daily life.

When you start out, it may be difficult to give up the high carb and processed foods that you are accustomed to eating. If you have made enough of an effort to purchase this cookbook, you are well on your way as you're mentally in the game. As with any lifestyle change, altering your relationship with food not only affects your choices in the grocery store, but your entire life. You will find that there may be unexpected obstacles that arise. However, if you find other like-minded people who are also on the same path, you will have a network to consult for any questions or suggestions on how to make the transition that much smoother.

One helpful step to encourage you to keep true to the Keto diet is to go through your fridge, freezer, and pantry to rid yourself of the foods you are not going to be eating any longer. A good suggestion is to donate these items to your local food bank so that it does not go to waste. You will also feel good about helping others in your community.

This step is also helpful because you're seeing what you have on hand, so that you do not go and purchase any unnecessary items, and use what you have in the recipes that follow.

The main steps in making sure that you do not falter are to educate yourself on the foods that you are allowed to eat, and the ones to avoid. Luckily, we have everything that you need to get started with these steps in the next two chapters. Read on!

Chapter 2: Keto Diet Food Choices

It cannot be stressed enough that you are going to need to read the labels for the products that you currently own, and the ones that you are going to buy in the future. Many items that are labeled as healthy alternatives, have additives that you are not going to want to consume to be true to your new diet.

As a general rule, if an item comes prepackaged, pay attention to the number of carbs that are included. Everyone has a different idea of what low carb is, especially when the typical American eats such much!

Don't worry so much about leaving your favorite comfort foods, because there are many renditions of your favorite snacks and recipes made healthier for you, and most of them taste just the same or better! You will find many classics in this recipe book. As you get further into your Keto experience, you will learn how to make your grandmother's yummy recipes by converting them Keto style!

You might even be surprised by some of the recipes in this book which include pizza, chips, fries, and even desserts!

The following is a listing of the foods you are going to want to incorporate into your diet and the ones you are going to cut out.

What is Included in a Balanced Keto Diet

For most people, you are going to want to stay below 20 net carbs within one day. This will keep your body in ketosis, and you will be successfully following the Keto diet. Here is an easy to follow list of the food groups and some examples of what you will be enjoying.

- *Eggs*: this is the most versatile item on the list because you can have eggs in any form that you wish.

- *Vegetables*: there is a wide variety of vegetables that you can eat. You will mainly stick to the greens that grow above the ground such as broccoli, avocado, cauliflower, spinach, and kale.

- *Seafood and fish*: these are an excellent source of fats and include items such as shrimp, lobster, and fatty fish such as salmon, tuna and mackerel.

- *Meat*: stick to the unprocessed cuts to keep within the guidelines of the Keto diet. You can eat poultry, beef, and lamb as they are high in the healthy fats and proteins your body needs. Yes, this also includes bacon!

- *Dairy*: the items that are high in macros such as full fat cream, butter, and hard cheese. You won't be able to have all dairy items, as you will read below.

- *Berries*: the best ones to have in your diet are blackberries, blueberries, raspberries, and strawberries.

- *Seeds and Nuts*: the most popular are almond, sunflower seeds, pecans, macadamia, and walnuts. Be careful to eat the correct amount as the macros can add up if you are using nuts as a snack.

- *Sweeteners*: these are substitutes that are used in place of traditional sugar. Stevia and Erythritol are the types that are used in this cookbook as they have the highest benefit to your health and they contain no carbs or fat.

- *Fatty dressings and oils*: coconut oil is going to be your new friend on the Keto diet as there are many health benefits including being high in fat. You can also have high-fat salad dressings.

- *Wine*: a glass of wine is acceptable in small amounts.

- *Coffee*: as long as you use a sweetener in your coffee, it is on the good list. If you enjoy milk in your coffee, switch to cream instead. Another alternative to boost your fat intake is to combine coconut oil and butter in your coffee. This is called Bulletproof Coffee! It is an excellent way to wake up in the morning.

- *Tea*: black, green and herbal teas are excellent on the Keto diet, as long as you use the sweeteners instead. Also the same as coffee, if you enjoy milk in your tea, cream is a better alternative.

As a note with the coffee and tea, if you are finding you have reached a plateau in your weight loss efforts, eliminate the cream or substitute the Bulletproof Coffee for a standard cup of Joe.

What Foods to Avoid for Optimum Results

Going back to reading the labels, steer clear of any items that include the words starch, dextrose, maltodextrin and of course sugar or cane syrup. These are all items you are going to be cutting out of your diet moving forward.

- *Milk*: the sugars contained in milk makes it extremely high in carbs. There are other more healthy alternatives that you will find out in these recipes.

- *Whole Fruits*: bananas, oranges, apples, and peaches are on this list. This also includes dried fruits as they contain high amounts of sugar.

- *Whole Grains*: keto is a gluten-free diet, as gluten is simple carbohydrates. This also includes items such as cereal, corn, and rice.

- *Processed foods*: other than the additives that are included, these are generally based on sugars and carbs, and you will find much more satisfying foods on the Keto diet.

- *Sugars*: as a general rule, all sugar is going to be eliminated as these will take you out of ketosis. These include agave, maple syrup, and honey as well.

As said before, don't worry so much about what you are cutting out of your diet. There is a multitude of options that are available on the Keto diet that are wholesome and satisfying! Many recipes taste the same or better, and will keep you on the straight track to bettering your overall health!

165

And speaking about health, the next chapter talks about the health benefits that you can experience on the Keto diet. But first, take a look at the shopping list which has the most common ingredients that you will find in this cookbook.

Shopping List

If you are able to buy these items in bulk, it will end up saving you more money as you incorporate the Keto diet. Also, look for sale items or even online shopping networks, to lower your costs to keep Keto cost effective for you. Remember to look at the labels and be sure to get sugar free, gluten free and unsweetened products to ensure that you are not buying anything that is not Keto.

This is a list of the most common ingredients that are used in Keto, and specifically in this cookbook that you will want to keep in stock in your pantry and fridge:

Meats

bacon
beef steak
canned chicken
canned tuna
chicken breast

chicken
drumsticks
flat iron steak
ground beef
ground pork

ground sausage
ground turkey
ham
sirloin *steak*

Dairy

almond butter
almond milk
butter
coconut milk

eggs
heavy cream
heavy whipping cream

mayonnaise
sour cream

Dry Goods

almond flour
almonds
chocolate chips
coconut flakes
coconut flour

dark chocolate
Erythritol
sweetener
flax meal
liquid Stevia

Swerve
sweetener
walnuts

Vegetables

asparagus spears
avocado
bell peppers
blueberries
broccoli
cabbage
carrots
cauliflower

celery stalks
chipotle peppers
cucumbers
green beans
kale
leek
lettuce

mixed green
salad
mushrooms
radishes
spinach
tomatoes
turnips
zucchini

Dressings and Oils

Apple cider
vinegar
avocado oil
beef stock
chicken broth

coconut oil
coconut oil spray
lemon juice
lime juice
olive oil

tamari sauce
toasted sesame
oil

Spices

almond extract
baking powder
baking soda
basil
celery salt
celery seeds
chives
cilantro

dill
fennel seeds
garlic cloves
garlic powder
garlic salt
ginger
ground
cardamom

ground
cinnamon
ground
coriander
ground cumin
Italian seasoning
mustard
nutmeg

167

onion powder
oregano
paprika powder
parsley
pepper
red pepper
flakes
rosemary
salt
thyme
turmeric
vanilla extract

Nutritional Information Note for this cookbook

Nutritional information for the recipes provided is an approximate only. And substitutions that you use will alter the nutritional values and need to be personally researched to stay on track with the Keto diet. As such we cannot guarantee the complete accuracy of the nutritional information given for any recipe in this cookbook. Erythritol carbs are not included in the net carb counts as it has been shown not to impact blood sugar. The method that net carbs are calculated is the total amount of carbs minus the fiber.

Chapter 3: Health Benefits of the Keto Diet

Overall Health

There are benefits of the Keto diet that is hard to argue with as many people see the benefits quickly. It is why it has been so successful for millions of people, but they affect people differently.

Weight Loss

The result of the shift from eating the typical high-carb and fatty diet in America to eating a low-carb high-fat diet, is that you will feel more satisfied from making the switch.

This is due to the high amount of fats that are present in the Keto diet, and these are a powerful energy source for the body. Your body is left more satisfied, and in return, you will see your energy levels soar and be able to keep you more focused throughout the day. This also reduces the sugar crashes experienced prior because sugar consumption is eliminated.

This leads to the main advantage that most people will notice is weight loss, and conclusions from several medical studies states it is a healthy way of doing so. The reasoning for this is most of the weight loss is actually water weight due to the carbs being expended in the liver. Most people see the results quickly which keeps them motivated to keep going towards their personal goals.

Your body becomes a fat burning machine when your insulin

levels are extremely low, which makes the body creates ketones. This, in turn, makes the body turn to the fat that is stored in your body to burn for energy. There also have been studies done to prove that your lean body mass is protected during this weight loss process, which is a giant plus!

Diabetes

As stated, some people shouldn't go on the Keto diet, and if you should have Type 1 Diabetes, then you need to find another avenue. Consult your doctor for other options as the Keto diet may lower your blood sugar levels too low because of your dependency on insulin.

Also, if you are on insulin medication for Diabetes, pay attention before beginning the Keto diet, as the medication may not react appropriately to the desired lifestyle change.

As for the patients with Type 2 Diabetes, studies show that the Keto diet helps to improve your HbA1c levels. However, even this lifestyle change should be done under the direction of an expert because it can also lower your sugar levels too much, resulting in hypoglycemia! Usually, this happens when you are on a medication, which reduces your blood pressure.

The benefit that most Type 2 Diabetes sufferers will notice, is that it helps the body to keep glucose levels at a more healthy level. This is due to the elimination of the sudden spikes in blood sugar from the lower amount of carbs consumed. This results in less insulin needed by these patients.

Chapter 4: Meal Preparation and Proper Storage

The Benefits of Meal Prepping

There are many advantages to meal prepping that you would not necessarily think about. The main benefits to meal prepping, are that you are going to save a lot of time and money! Now, everyone needs more of both of those! Read more about how to easy implement this technique into your Keto lifestyle.

How to Get Started

When you plan your meals out ahead of time, you will need to create a shopping list. This is so you stay within your budget, and not buy unnecessary items that may go bad in your fridge before you have a chance to use them. It also gives you a chance to see what you have on hand, and it may be the case that you don't need to go shopping at all.

When you'll go to the store, it will best to refrain from going down the aisles that most tempted you in your old way of life, such as the cookie aisle! The longer you stay true to the diet, you will find that you will pass them right by because there will be no need for sugary snacks. Also, as a general rule, do not shop while you are hungry! This method will also help in keeping you within your budget and to stay on track with your new lifestyle. Also, the longer you are on the Keto diet, hunger will not be much of an issue.

Because you will be cooking the meals ahead of time and bringing your meals with you to the office or the gym, you will not be tempted to pick up the snacks and meals that you used to when you are out and about. And since you will already have your meals with you, the temptation to go out to a restaurant with your co-workers will be lessened, and you will be able to stick to your new lifestyle choice more easily.

Any of these recipes can easily be doubled or even tripled to help keep you and your family on course, and it will save you time from having to cook meals throughout the day. There are proper storage and heating techniques that we will talk about in the next section that will help you with your leftovers.

Storage and Reheating of Your Meals

Many of these recipes can be stored either on the counter, fridge or freezer to be easily eaten when the hunger pangs strike. You will need to acquire some stock in zip lock bags, and lidded tubs to make sure you are able to store your leftovers and made-ahead meals properly.

Also, if you are really serious and do not have a lot of storage space, consider purchasing a FoodSaver. It's a small expense up front, but you will be able to pack more food into the space you have, your meals and snacks will stay fresher for longer, and it minimizes the risk of freezer burn. The FoodSaver works by simply sucking out all the air in your ziplock bags, creating the space that you will need.

As for any meats or vegetables that you store in the refrigerator or freezer, make sure that you label with the item name and date that you packed the leftovers. This will eliminate any guesswork as to when they were stored which will make sure that you do not thaw out food, that is not good for you anymore.

If you are going to store your snacks on the counter, keep them in an air-tight container as they will stay longer. As a note, the cookies and granola bars will need to be eaten within five days if stored on the counter. If you keep them in the refrigerator, they will keep up to a week, and if you freeze them, they will last up to a month.

Storing your Keto meals in the freezer or the refrigerator are just as easy! Simply, put them in a sealed container or throw them into a ziplock plastic bag. If you are storing them in the freezer, be sure to put them in a freezer safe container or zip lock bag. Also, remove any excess air ahead of time.

Ensure your meals and snacks are cooled entirely beforehand. This will prevent moisture from creating condensation in your storage containers and bags, keeping your meals fresher.

Whenever you are ready to eat your premade meals and leftovers, you can put them back into the oven to heat them, or throw them into the microwave. All other specific storing tips for the recipes will be found in the individual recipes themselves.

Most of the recipes will need to be consumed within a week before they go sour. If there are meals that you know you are not going to be able to eat before that time, you can freeze them!

Now that we have gotten through all the education and background of the Keto diet let us get to the best part – cooking your new and exciting meals and snacks in your kitchen.

Enjoy!

Chapter 5: Breakfast Recipes

Almond Butter Shake

Get your morning started right with this fantastic boost in energy that takes just 5 minutes to make.

Total Prep & Cooking Time: 5 minutes
Level: Beginner
Makes: 1 Shake
Protein: 19 grams
Net Carbs: 6 grams
Fat: 27 grams
Sugar: 0 grams
Calories: 326

What you need:

1 1/2 cups almond milk, unsweetened
2 tbs almond butter
1/2 tbs ground cinnamon
2 tbs flax meal
1/8 tsp almond extract, sugar-free
15 drops liquid Stevia
1/8 tsp salt
6 ice cubes

Steps:

1. Using a blender, combine all the listed ingredients and pulse for approximately 45 seconds.
2. Serve immediately and enjoy!

Bacon & Egg Fat Bomb

Healthy packed breakfast fat bombs that are guaranteed to satisfy you throughout the morning.

Total Prep & Cooking Time: 50 minutes
Level: Beginner
Makes: 3 Fat Bombs
Protein: 2 grams
Net Carbs: 0.1 grams
Fat: 13 grams
Sugar: 0 grams
Calories: 127

What you need:

1 large egg
12 cups of cold water, separated
1/4 tsp salt
3 tsp mayonnaise, sugar-free
1/8 cup butter
2 slices bacon
1/8 tsp pepper

Steps:

1. Fill a pot with 6 cups of the cold water and the eggs.
2. Set the timer for 7 minutes once the water starts to boil.
3. When the time has passed, drain the water and pour the remaining 6 cups of cold water on the eggs to halt the heating process.
4. Once cooled, peel the eggs and place in a dish with the butter, pepper, mayonnaise, and salt, whisking until combined.
5. Refrigerate for approximately half an hour.
6. Heat the bacon in a skillet until crispy and brown. Place on a plate with paper towels.
7. Crumble the bacon once cooled onto a small plate and remove the eggs from the fridge.
8. Scoop out small balls and cover entirely in the bacon bits, and serve immediately.

Belgium Waffles

Take yourself back to childhood with this classic breakfast which is a little taste of heaven.

Total Prep & Cooking Time: 10 minutes
Level: Beginner
Makes: 1 Helping (3 small waffles)
Protein: 4 grams
Net Carbs: 1 gram
Fat: 8 grams
Sugar: 0 grams
Calories: 81

What you need:

1 large egg
4 tsp almond butter, softened
1/4 tsp baking powder, gluten-free
2 tbs almond flour
1/8 tsp baking soda
1 tsp lemon juice
1/8 tsp salt

coconut oil spray
waffle maker

Steps:

1. Use a whisk to fully beat the egg in a dish and mix with the almond butter until combined.
2. Stir the salt, baking powder, and almond flour into the mixture until creamy.
3. Turn the waffle maker to high and spray with coconut oil.
4. Just before you transfer the batter, completely whisk in the lemon juice and baking soda into the mixture.
5. Cook the waffles to your desired crispness and serve immediately.

Variation Tips:
- If you want to add a bit of sweetness to the waffle, add 1 tablespoon of confectioner Swerve to the batter or top your waffles with a dusting.

Blueberry Muffins

Get your antioxidant and energy filled fat boost from these moist and delicious muffins.

Total Prep & Cooking Time: 30 minutes
Level: Beginner
Makes: 6 Muffins
Protein: 7 grams
Net Carbs: 3 grams
Fat: 19 grams
Sugar: 2 grams
Calories: 217

What you need:

1/3 cup blueberries
3/4 tsp baking powder, gluten-free
1 1/4 cup almond flour, blanched
2 1/2 tbs coconut oil, melted
1/4 cup Erythritol sweetener, granulated
2 1/2 tbs almond milk, unsweetened

1/8 tsp salt

2 large eggs

1/4 tsp vanilla extract, sugar-free

Steps:

1. Set the stove to heat at 350° Fahrenheit. Use baking or non-stick muffin liners to layer the cupcake cups.
2. In a big dish, blend the Erythritol, baking powder, salt, and almond flour until combined.
3. Whisk in the almond milk, eggs, melted coconut oil, and vanilla extract until a creamy consistency.
4. Carefully stir the blueberries in the batter with a rubber scraper.
5. Evenly empty into the baking cups and heat for 20 minutes.
6. Enjoy immediately.

Variation Tips:

- If you have a nut allergy, substitute the almond flour for sunflower seed meal, just know the muffins may have a slight green tint.
- You can use either fresh or frozen blueberries. If you opt for the frozen, do not thaw them ahead of time.

Breakfast Pizza

You might just want to have dinner for breakfast with this brilliantly filling pizza. Of course, you could always just make it at any time of the day.

Total Prep & Cooking Time: 45 minutes
Level: Intermediate
Makes: 10 Slices
Protein: 5 grams
Net Carbs: 3 grams
Fat: 8 grams
Sugar: 1 gram
Calories: 121

What you need:

For the crust:

6 large eggs whites
1/2 cup coconut flour
8 oz. coconut milk, unsweetened
2 tsp garlic powder

1 tsp onion powder
2 tsp Italian seasoning
1/2 tsp baking soda

For the toppings:

1 tbs extra-virgin olive oil
3 large eggs
1 tomato, sliced thinly
8 oz. baby spinach
1/2 tsp red pepper, flaked

Steps:

1. Set the stove to the temperature of 375° Fahrenheit to heat. Cover a large flat sheet with baking lining.
2. In a mixing dish, blend the coconut milk, egg whites, and coconut flour until combined.
3. Spice with Italian seasoning, garlic powder, and onion powder.
4. Spread the batter uniformly on the prepped flat sheet in a rectangle.
5. Heat for approximately 15 minutes until crisp and remove.
6. Reduce the stove temperature to 350° Fahrenheit.
7. While still warm, brush the olive oil onto the entire crust.
8. Layer the spinach and tomatoes on the crust. Break the eggs and pour on the top carefully. Finally, dust with the red pepper.
9. Heat for another 12 min. until the eggs are completely baked and remove.
10. Slice into 10 sections and serve warm.

Burrito Bowl

This is a burrito that does not even need the tortillas to deliver this nourishing low carb breakfast.

Total Prep & Cooking Time: 30 minutes
Level: Intermediate
Makes: 12 Fat Bombs
Protein: 14 grams
Net Carbs: 4 grams
Fat: 14 grams
Sugar: 2 grams
Calories: 299

What you need:

1/2 lb. ground beef, lean
3/4 cup water

1 cup cauliflower
2 tbs cilantro, chopped
1 tsp butter, melted
3 large eggs
1/4 tsp salt
3 tsp taco seasoning
1/8 tsp pepper

Steps:

1. Split the cauliflower into pieces and place in a food blender. Pulse for approximately 60 seconds until crumbly.
2. Heat the cauliflower in a saucepan for about 5 minutes as it becomes tender. Remove from heat.
3. Spoon the cauliflower into a tea towel and wring to eliminate the excess water. Repeat this step as many times as necessary to ensure the liquid has been removed. Put aside.
4. In another dish, beat the eggs and butter together and set to the side.
5. Use a skillet to brown the ground beef for approximately 7 minutes. Drain the fat and stir the water and taco seasoning into the meat.
6. Boil the water and reduce the heat. Allow to rest for approximately 3 additional minutes while simmering.
7. Section off the meat to one side of the pan. Pour the riced cauliflower into the clear area of the pan and sprinkle with the cilantro.
8. Heat and brown for approximately 4 minutes and press to the side of the pan to clear space for the egg mixture.
9. Prepare the eggs to your preference and then combine everything in the pan fully.
10. Spice with the seasons to your personal taste and serve.

Baking Tip:

- If you find that your skillet is not large enough to cook all the ingredients in one pan, use a separate frying pan as necessary.

Fluffy Pancakes

Bring an old tradition back into your kitchen with this Keto friendly version of pancakes that will remind you of the old-fashioned version.

Total Prep & Cooking Time: 30 minutes
Level: Beginner
Makes: 2 Pancakes
Protein: 4 grams
Net Carbs: 1 gram
Fat: 10 grams
Sugar: 0 grams
Calories: 118

What you need:

1/8 tsp baking powder, gluten-free
4 oz. almond flour
2 1/2 tsp almond milk, unsweetened
1/4 tsp vanilla extract, sugar-free
1 large egg
1 tbs coconut oil

Steps:

1. Melt the coconut oil in a skillet while mixing the batter.
2. Using a food blender, whip the baking powder, egg and almond milk for 20 seconds. Combine the almond flour and vanilla extract and continue to pulse for approximately 30 seconds.
3. Transfer half the batter to the hot skillet and flip over the pancake after about 60 seconds. Continue to flip until golden. Repeat for the remaining batter. Serve immediately.

Variation Tips:
- Top with healthy blueberries, crispy bacon or enjoy as is.
- Alternatively, you can use 2 1/2 teaspoons of heavy cream in place of the almond milk.

Home Fries

You do not have to give up your breakfast potatoes with this turnip alternative that tastes like the real thing.

Total Prep & Cooking Time: 20 minutes
Level: Beginner
Makes: 4 Helpings
Protein: 3 grams
Net Carbs: 4 grams
Fat: 6 grams
Sugar: 0 grams
Calories: 88

What you need:

1/2 tsp paprika powder
2 cups turnips, peeled and diced
1/4 tbs onion powder
3 slices bacon
1/2 tsp garlic powder
3 tsp olive oil
1/2 tsp salt
2 oz. parsley, chopped

1/2 tsp pepper

Steps:

1. In a large skillet, warm the olive oil.
2. In a dish, incorporate the seasonings of paprika powder, onion powder, and garlic powder and the turnips until completely covered.
3. When the oil is hot enough, heat the turnips for approximately 10 minutes while occasionally stirring.
4. Chop the bacon into small chunks and fry with the turnips for an additional 5 mins.
5. Garnish it with parsley and serve.

Variation Tip:
- You can mix and match the garnishes with pickles, olive oil or pine nuts.

Sausage Patties

No traditional breakfast would be complete without sausage patties. Packed with protein, these would be wonderful before your morning run.

Total Prep & Cooking Time: 20 minutes
Level: Beginner
Makes: 4 Patties
Protein: 25 grams
Net Carbs: 5.2 grams
Fat: 9 grams
Sugar: 1 gram
Calories: 272

What you need:

1/3 tsp onion powder
3/4 lb. ground pork
1/3 tsp salt
4 3/4 oz. mushrooms, chopped
1/3 tsp garlic powder
4 oz. kale, thinly sliced
1/8 tsp ground ginger

2 tbs coconut oil, separated
1/8 tsp nutmeg
2 garlic cloves, minced
1/4 tsp fennel seeds

Steps:

1. Melt 1 tablespoon of coconut oil in a skillet.
2. Put in the mushrooms, minced garlic and kale and stir fry for approximately 5 minutes and remove from heat.
3. In a dish, combine the ground pork, cooked vegetables, onion powder, garlic powder, nutmeg, and fennel seeds.
4. Divide into 4 sections and create patties by hand.
5. In the same skillet, pour a tablespoon of coconut oil and heat.
6. Fry the patties for approximately 2 minutes and turn over to brown the other side. Flip over as necessary to fully cook the meat in the middle of the patties.
7. Serve immediately and enjoy.

Variation Tip:

- You can choose to mix up the recipe using different meat or vegetables such as ground turkey or beef and spinach or bell peppers.

Tuna Omelet

Breakfast would not be complete without a healthy omelet to get your day started on the right foot.

Total Prep & Cooking Time: 15 minutes
Level: Beginner
Makes: 2 Omelets
Protein: 28 grams
Net Carbs: 4.9 grams
Fat: 18 grams
Sugar: 1 gram
Calories: 260

What you need:

2 tbs coconut oil
1 medium green bell pepper, deseeded and diced
2 1/2 oz. canned tuna, spring water and drained
1/4 tsp salt
6 large eggs
1/8 tsp pepper

Steps:

1. Melt the coconut oil in a small skillet and fry the green pepper for approximately 3 minutes. Remove from the burner.
2. Transfer the peppers into a dish and combine the tuna until fully together. Set to the side.
3. Beat the eggs, salt, and pepper in a separate dish as the coconut oil is melting in a small non-stick skillet.
4. Move the pan around to ensure the entire base is coated in oil and very hot.
5. Empty the beaten eggs into the skillet and use a rubber spatula to lift the edge of the cooked eggs in several areas to allow the uncooked eggs to heat.
6. Once there is a thin layer of cooked egg created, leave the pan on the heat for half a minute to fully set.
7. Scoop half of the peppers and tuna onto one side of the eggs. Use the rubber spatula to flip over the cooked eggs to create an omelet.
8. Press down lightly until the omelet naturally seals and after approximately 1 minute, move to a serving plate.
9. Repeat steps 4 through 8 with the second omelet.

Baking Tip:
- If you do not have a ton of time in the mornings, you can create the omelet filling the evening before and refrigerate in a lidded container.

Variation Tip:
- You may choose to garnish the top of the omelet with additional salt and pepper to taste or chopped chives.

Chapter 6: Lunch Recipes

Avocado Chicken Salad

Enjoy this colorful mix of the customary chicken salad that is low in carbs and high in potassium. Your heart will be thanking you.

Total Prep & Cooking Time: 15 minutes

Level: Beginner

Makes: 4 Helpings

Protein: 14 grams

Net Carbs: 0.4 grams

Fat: 2 grams

Sugar: 0 grams

Calories: 74

What you need:

12.5 oz. canned chicken, drained and shredded

1 large avocado

8 oz. cilantro, chopped

1/4 tsp salt
8 oz. celery, chopped
1/8 tsp pepper

Steps:

1. Mash the avocado using a food blender for approximately half a minute. Combine the chicken, salt, chopped cilantro, chopped celery, and pepper and pulse until incorporated.
2. Transfer to a serving plate and enjoy.

Variation Tip:
- Instead of canned chicken, you can use the same amount of rotisserie chicken. You can eat as is, place on a leaf of lettuce or a slice of low carb bread.

Burger Cabbage Stir Fry

This quick lunch dish is easy to whip up even in the morning so it can be brought with you to work.

Total Prep & Cooking Time: 20 minutes
Level: Beginner
Makes: 4 Helpings
Protein: 9 grams
Net Carbs: 1.5 grams
Fat: 8 grams
Sugar: 1 gram
Calories: 208

What you need:

1/4 tsp salt
5 oz. ground beef
1 tsp onion powder
8 oz. cabbage, sliced

1 clove garlic, minced

2 tbs coconut oil

1/8 tsp pepper

Steps:

1. In a big skillet, combine the bacon and beef and brown for approximately 7 minutes.
2. Then fry the minced garlic, chopped cabbage and onion powder with the meat for about 2 additional minutes.
3. Serve warm after seasoning with pepper and salt.

Baking Tip:

- For this stir fry, you can also use a wok instead of the skillet.

Cauliflower Fried Rice

You will fall in love with this rendition of fried rice which will also go together as a side for any meal.

Total Prep & Cooking Time: 15 minutes
Makes: 4 Helpings
Protein: 4 grams
Net Carb: 5 grams
Fat: 8 grams
Sugar: 0 grams
Calories: 114

What you need:

2 tbs butter
12 oz. riced cauliflower, florets
1 tbs onion powder
2 cloves garlic, crushed
1 large egg, beaten
2 tbs tamari sauce, gluten-free
1 tsp toasted sesame oil

Steps:

1. Using a food blender, pulse the cauliflower florets for about 1 minute on high until crumbly.
2. Heat the cauliflower in a saucepan for approximately 5 minutes and remove from the heat.
3. Spoon the cauliflower into a tea towel and twist to remove moisture. Repeat this step multiple times to make sure most of the water has been removed.
4. For 5 mins., brown the cauliflower with hot butter.
5. Add in the garlic and onion powder, stirring occasionally for one minute.
6. Incorporate the beaten egg into the skillet and continuously stir for approximately 2 additional minutes. Remove from heat.
7. Finally, season with the tamari sauce and toasted sesame oil and serve warm.

Variation Tips:

- If you do not want to cook with butter, you can alternatively use 2 tablespoons of olive oil, ghee or coconut oil.
- If you want to save time ricing the cauliflower, you can use frozen premade riced cauliflower in this recipe.
- For variety, you can add 1/4 cup of diced carrots.

Cobb Salad

This flavorful easy to make salad can be done in advance and put into a container to bring with you to work or the gym.

Total Prep & Cooking Time: 30 minutes
Level: Beginner
Makes: 1 Salad
Protein: 24 grams
Net Carbs: 4.7 grams
Fat: 18 grams
Sugar: 2 grams
Calories: 337

What you need:

4 cherry tomatoes
3/4 cup avocado
1 large egg
2 cups mixed green salad

1/4 cup cooked bacon, crumbled

2 oz. chicken breast, shredded

4 cups cold water

1 tbs coconut oil, melted

Steps:

1. Fill a saucepan with 2 cups of the cold water and the egg.
2. Once the water starts to boil, set a timer for 7 minutes.
3. When the timer goes off, drain the water and pour the remaining 2 cups of cold water on the egg to cool.
4. Once it can be handled, peel the egg and slice into large chunks.
5. Brown the bacon in a skillet with the coconut oil until crispy. Set on a paper towel covered plate.
6. Dice the avocado and tomatoes.
7. In a bowl, empty the mixed greens and combine the chicken. Crush the bacon into the salad dish.
8. Finally, transfer the diced avocado, tomatoes and egg to the top. Serve immediately.

Variation Tip:

- Drizzle one tablespoon of ranch dressing on top of your salad. This will add approximately 8 grams of fat and 73 calories.

Egg Salad

Whip this egg salad up in no time and enjoy the fantastic boost in energy from this fat bomb.

Total Prep & Cooking Time: 15 minutes
Level: Beginner
Makes: 2 Helpings
Protein: 6 grams
Net Carbs: 1 gram
Fat: 28 grams
Sugar: 1 gram
Calories: 260

What you need:

3 tbs mayonnaise, sugar-free
1/4 cup celery, chopped
2 large eggs, hardboiled and yolks separated.
1/2 tsp mustard

3 tbs red bell pepper, chopped
1/4 tsp salt
3 tbs broccoli, riced
1/4 tsp pepper
2 tbs mushroom, chopped
1/4 tsp paprika
4 cups cold water

Steps:

1. Fill a saucepan with the eggs and 2 cups of the cold water.
2. When the water begins to boil, set a timer for 7 minutes.
3. After the time has passed, drain the water and empty the remaining 2 cups of cold water over the eggs.
4. Once they can be handled, peel the eggs and remove the yolks. Chop the egg whites and leave to the side.
5. In a large dish, blend the mayonnaise, mustard, salt and egg yolks.
6. Combine the chopped celery, bell pepper, broccoli, and mushroom.
7. Finally, integrate the egg whites, pepper and paprika until combined fully.

Hamburger Salad

You will not be missing the bun when you bite into this delicious salad that you will want to have more than once a week.

Total Prep & Cooking Time: 20 minutes
Level: Beginner
Makes: 4 Helpings
Protein: 16 grams
Net Carbs: 2 grams
Fat: 27 grams
Sugar: 1 gram
Calories: 330

What you need:

For the salad:

3/4 lb. ground beef
1/2 tsp salt
3/4 cup romaine lettuce
1/8 tsp pepper
3/4 cup tomatoes, chopped

1/3 cup pickles, diced
2 tbs coconut oil

For the dressing:

1/3 cup mayonnaise, sugar-free
4 tsp pickles, diced
1 1/2 tsp mustard
2/3 tsp white vinegar
1/3 tsp paprika powder
3 tsp Erythritol sweetener, confectioner

Steps:

1. In a large skillet, melt the coconut oil. Brown the ground beef for approximately 7 minutes and season with salt and add some pepper.
2. In a food blender, cream the mayonnaise, pickles, mustard, vinegar, paprika, and Erythritol. Move to the refrigerator until ready to serve.
3. In a salad bowl, layer the romaine lettuce, pickles, and tomatoes. Empty the browned beef in the bowl and toss.
4. Top with the salad dressing and enjoy!

Roasted Veggie Masala

This popular Indian flavored vegetable sheet pan dish will be a delectable addition to your Keto diet.

Total Prep & Cooking Time: 30 minutes
Level: Intermediate
Makes: 4 Helpings
Protein: 3 grams
Net Carbs: 6 grams
Fat: 7 grams
Sugar: 0 grams
Calories: 105

What you need:

8 oz. cauliflower
1/2 tsp chili powder
6 oz. green beans, sliced
1/4 tsp turmeric
4 oz. mushrooms, quartered

1/4 tsp garam masala

8 oz. tomato puree

1 clove garlic, minced

2 tbs olive oil

1/4 tsp salt

2 tsp fresh ginger, minced

1/8 tsp pepper

Steps:

1. Set your stove to preheat to the temperature of 400° Fahrenheit. Cover a flat sheet with tin foil and set aside.
2. Slice the green beans and mushrooms. Mince the ginger and garlic and set to the side.
3. In a glass bowl, whisk the chili powder, turmeric, garam masala, and olive oil until blended.
4. Combine the minced ginger, garlic and tomato puree until mixed together well. Then toss the green beans and mushrooms in the mixture, coating fully.
5. Transfer to the prepped flat sheet in one layer and sprinkle the salt and pepper on top.
6. Heat in the stove for 20 minutes and serve immediately.

Baking Tips:

- Instead of baking in the stove, you can stir fry the vegetables in a wok or large non-stick skillet with the minced garlic and ginger on high heat. After approximately 10 minutes, reduce the heat to medium. Pour the spices and tomato puree into the skillet, stir and simmer for an additional 5 minutes. Before serving, season with pepper and salt.

- If garam masala is not available, you can make your own! Simply add 1/16 teaspoon allspice and 3/16 teaspoon cumin seasonings.

Variation Tips:
- Garnish options for this dish are 2 tablespoons of chopped cilantro or 1 tablespoon of sriracha.
- Alternatively, you can use ghee or melted butter in place of the 2 tablespoons of olive oil.

Spicy Cauliflower Turkey

This moist dish will keep you satisfied throughout the day and have you coming back for seconds at dinnertime.

Total Prep & Cooking Time: 25 minutes
Level: Beginner
Makes: 4 Helpings
Protein: 23 grams
Net Carbs: 4.4 grams
Fat: 24 grams
Sugar: 0 grams
Calories: 310

What you need:

3/4 tsp salt
12 oz. ground turkey
3/4 tbs mustard
1 2/3 cups cauliflower
3/4 tsp pepper

2 tbs coconut oil

3/4 tsp thyme

1 tsp onion powder

3/4 tsp salt

2 cloves garlic

3/4 tsp garlic powder

1 2/3 cups coconut milk, full fat

3/4 tsp celery salt

Steps:

1. Pulse the cauliflower florets in a food blender for approximately 1 minute on high until crumbly.
2. Heat the cauliflower in a saucepan.
3. Scoop the cauliflower into a tea towel and twist to remove the moisture, repeating as necessary until as much of the water is removed as possible.
4. Heat a large pot and melt the coconut oil.
5. Mince the garlic and pour into the hot pot to simmer for approximately 2 minutes.
6. Combine the ground turkey to the garlic and brown for about 7 minutes, stirring with a wooden scraper to break up the meat.
7. Blend the riced cauliflower, salt, thyme, garlic powder, celery salt, mustard, and pepper with the meat until combined.
8. Reduce the temperature and finally add the coconut milk. Simmer for approximately 6 additional minutes.
9. Serve hot and enjoy!

Variation Tips:
- If you continue to reduce the dish by half and it will become thicker and can be served as a dip at your next party.

- Alternatively, you can use ground pork, lamb or beef with this recipe. You can also add other vegetables such as broccoli.
- Optional garnishes include bacon, cherry tomatoes, hot sauce or jalapenos.

Spinach & Ham Quiche

When you want a wholesome lunch that is ready in half an hour, this will surely fit the bill.

Total Prep & Cooking Time: 30 minutes
Level: Beginner
Makes: 2 Quiches
Protein: 20 grams
Net Carbs: 2 grams
Fat: 13 grams
Sugar: 1 gram
Calories: 210

What you need:

1/4 cup coconut milk
3 large eggs, whisked
1/2 tsp baking powder, gluten-free
4 slices of ham, diced
12 oz. spinach, chopped

1/8 tsp pepper
4 oz. leek, chopped
1/4 tsp salt
Coconut oil spray

Steps:

1. Set your stove to preheat to the temperature of 350° Fahrenheit. Spray 2 mini tart or quiche pans with coconut oil.
2. In a large glass bowl, blend the ham, leek, salt, spinach, eggs, pepper, coconut milk, and baking powder until incorporated fully.
3. Empty evenly into the quiche pans and heat for 15 minutes in the stove.
4. Remove and enjoy warm.

Turkey Burger Patties

You do not have to give up having heart healthy burgers while choosing to live a better life.

Total Prep & Cooking Time: 30 minutes
Level: Beginner
Makes: 4 Patties
Protein: 11 grams
Net Carbs: 1 gram
Fat: 8 grams
Sugar: 1 gram
Calories: 117

What you need:

1/2 tsp oregano seasoning
3 tsp olive oil
1/2 tsp basil seasoning
8 oz. zucchini, grated
1/4 tsp salt
8 oz. ground turkey, lean
1/8 tsp red pepper flakes
1 clove garlic, minced
1/8 tsp pepper
1 tsp parsley seasoning

1/4 tsp onion powder

Steps:

1. In a large dish, blend the ground turkey, oregano, basil, zucchini, salt, red pepper, garlic, parsley, pepper, and onion powder until completely combined.
2. Divide the meat into 4 sections and create patties by hand.
3. Using a large skillet, heat olive oil. Once the skillet is hot, transfer the patties to the fry for approximately 5 minutes and then flip to the other side.
4. Fry for an additional 5 minutes until cooked fully.
5. Serve warm and enjoy!

Chapter 7: Snack Recipes

Bacon Wrapped Avocado

This quick fried snack is going to have you filling up on the nutrients and fats that your body craves.

Total Prep & Cooking Time: 30 minutes
Level: Beginner
Makes: 3 Helpings (2 wraps per serving)
Protein: 15 grams
Net Carbs: 1.8 grams
Fat: 21 grams
Sugar: 0 grams
Calories: 139

What you need:

1 avocado, peeled and pitted
6 strips bacon
1 tbs butter

Steps:

1. Slice the avocado into 6 individual wedges.
2. Wrap one slice of bacon around the avocado wedge and repeat for all pieces.
3. Soften the butter in a non-stick skillet and transfer the wedges to the hot butter with the end of the bacon on the base of the pan. This will prevent the bacon from coming apart from the wedge.
4. Cook for approximately 3 minutes on each side, and move to a paper towel covered plate.
5. Serve while still hot and enjoy!

Baking Tip:
- Do not use an avocado that is mushy or overripe as it will crumble while wrapping with the bacon.

Variation Tip:
- You can also substitute asparagus instead of the avocado.

Chicken Tenders

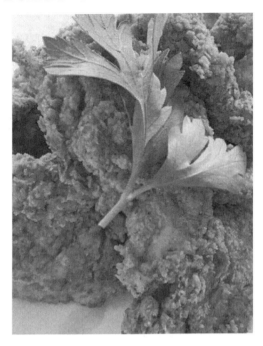

Move over chicken nuggets! These are a much more improved alternative to your childhood snack.

Total Prep & Cooking Time: 20 minutes
Level: Beginner
Makes: 2 Helpings (3 tenders per serving)
Protein: 26 grams
Net Carbs: 0.7 grams
Fat: 9 grams
Sugar: 0 grams
Calories: 220

What you need:

1/2 cup coconut oil
8 oz. chicken breast tenderloins

1 tsp pepper, separated

8 oz. almond flour

1 tsp salt, separated

4 oz. heavy whipping cream

1 large egg

Steps:

1. In a large dish, blend the egg and heavy whipping cream with the 1/2 teaspoon of pepper and 1/2 teaspoon of salt.
2. Soak the chicken pieces in the blend for approximately 10 minutes.
3. Using a skillet, melt the coconut oil.
4. Pour the almond flour onto a small bowl and season with the remaining 1/2 teaspoon of pepper and 1/2 teaspoon of salt.
5. Remove the individual pieces of chicken and coat both sides with the almond flour. Set a 13 x 9-inch glass dish to the side.
6. Transfer the chicken to the hot coconut oil and fry for approximately 3 minutes on the side.
7. Serve hot and enjoy!

Baking Tip:

- You can also bake these in the oven if you wish. Set the stove to 425° Fahrenheit and prepare a flat sheet with a heavy coating of olive oil. Follow the steps for breading the chicken tenders and place on the prepped sheet. Heat for 10 minutes, flip them and continue to heat for another 10 mins. Note: they will not be as crispy as when they are fried.

Chocolate Brownie Cookies

Chewy and chocolaty, you cannot go wrong with this midday or afternoon snack to cure your sweet tooth cravings.

Total Prep & Cooking Time: 25 minutes
Level: Beginner
Makes: 6 Cookies
Protein: 2 grams
Net Carbs: 1.2 grams
Fat: 5 grams
Sugar: 0 grams
Calories: 53

What you need:

1 egg, beaten
2 1/3 tbs cocoa powder
1 oz. cream cheese softened
2 oz. Swerve sweetener
1/3 tsp baking powder
2 tbs mini dark chocolate chips, unsweetened

Steps:

1. Set your stove to preheat to the temperature of 350° Fahrenheit. Cover a flat sheet with baking lining and set to the side.
2. In a food blender, whip the cream cheese, Swerve, baking powder, cocoa powder, and egg until all lumps are removed.
3. Use a rubber scraper to stir in 1 tablespoon of the mini chocolate chips.
4. Spoon out the dough onto the prepped pan in small mounds. Press the tops to flatten and dust with the remaining tablespoon of mini chocolate chips.
5. Heat in the stove for approximately 12 minutes and remove to the counter.
6. Wait about 10 minutes before removing from the cookie sheet and enjoy!

Coleslaw Salad

This is a simple salad recipe that will be an easy, quick snack when you need it most.

Total Prep & Cooking Time: 10 minutes
Level: Beginner
Makes: 4 Helpings
Protein: 1 gram
Net Carbs: 1.5 grams
Fat: 15 grams
Sugar: 0 grams
Calories: 134

What you need:

1 tsp mustard
14 oz. coleslaw mix
1 tsp garlic salt
8 oz. mayonnaise, sugar-free
1 tsp black pepper
2 tbs heavy cream
1 tsp chives

Steps:

1. Pulse the prepared coleslaw in a food blender for approximately half a minute to break up the large pieces.
2. Transfer the chopped coleslaw to a serving dish.
3. Combine the mustard, heavy cream, pepper, chives, mayonnaise, and garlic salt until creamy.
4. Pour the dressing into the serving dish and toss the coleslaw until completely mixed.
5. Serve immediately.

Variation Tips:

- If you prefer sweet coleslaw, blend 1 tablespoon of Swerve to the dressing or chop a tomato and add to the serving bowl with the coleslaw mix.

Crisp Garlic Pickles

When you want something crunchy, there is nothing much like a crispy pickle with a punch to get you through the afternoon.

Total Prep & Cooking Time: 10 minutes (plus marinating time: 2 days)
Level: Beginner
Makes: 4 Helpings
Protein: 0 grams
Net Carbs: 0 grams
Fat: 0 grams
Calories: 5

What you need:

1/4 tsp black peppercorns, whole
8 oz. pickling cucumbers
1/2 tsp dill
4 oz. apple cider vinegar
1/4 tsp mustard seeds

4 oz. water

1/2 tbs pickling salt

1 1/2 cloves garlic, peeled

Steps:

1. Cut the cucumbers into thick wedges or slices.
2. In a large dish, mix all the ingredients and move to a mason jar.
3. Refrigerate for 2 full days before serving, and they will keep for up to one month.

Granola Bars

This sweet and crunchy snack is easily transportable and will kick any slag in energy that you may have.

Total Prep & Cooking Time: 1 hour 30 minutes
Level: Intermediate
Makes: 4 Bars
Protein: 4 grams
Net Carbs: 3.6 grams
Fat: 16 grams
Sugar: 1 gram
Calories: 176

What you need:

1/8 cup chocolate chips, Stevia sweetened
2 1/2 oz. almonds, raw and chopped
1 tsp flax seeds
2 1/2 oz. coconut flakes, unsweetened
4 tsp Swerve sweetener, confectioner

2 1/2 oz. almonds, sliced
1 tbs coconut oil
2/3 tbs almond butter
1/4 tsp salt

Steps:

1. Set the oven to heat at 375° Fahrenheit. Layer a piece of baking lining over a small pan, with plenty left over each of the sides. Prepare three small flat sheets with baking paper.
2. Spread the chopped almonds on 1 of the prepped sheets and heat for about 10 minutes. Place on the counter.
3. Pour the slivered almonds on the second prepped sheet and heat for approximately 4 minutes. Remove to the counter.
4. On the last prepped sheet, scatter the coconut flakes and heat for about 3 minutes. Place with the other prepped sheets on the counter.
5. Adjust the temperature to 350° Fahrenheit.
6. In a saucepan, dissolve the coconut oil and almond butter.
7. In a big dish, whip the egg and Swerve.
8. Transfer the toasted almonds and coconut and combine fully.
9. With a rubber scraper, incorporate the salt and chocolate chips into the batter.
10. Evenly press the batter into the prepped 8-inch pan making sure all air is out of the batter.
11. Heat for approximately 15 minutes and remove to the counter to cool for at least half an hour.
12. Cut into 4 even pieces and serve.

Baking Tip:

- The coconut needs to be tightly packed when measuring to ensure the proper amount.

Variation Tip:

- Alternatively, you can use dairy-free unsweetened chocolate in this recipe.

Mashed Cauliflower

Missing potatoes? You will not anymore with this brilliant substitution which tastes so good; you will not be able to taste the difference.

Total Prep & Cooking Time: 25 minutes
Level: Beginner
Makes: 4 Helpings
Protein: 4 grams
Net Carbs: 6 grams
Fat: 13 grams
Sugar: 0 grams
Calories: 227

What you need:

1/2 cup chives, chopped
3 cups cauliflower

1 tsp salt
2 tbs olive oil
1/4 cup parsley
3 cloves garlic, chopped
1 tsp pepper
8 oz. sour cream
6 cups of water

Steps:

1. Boil the water in a large pot and sauté the cauliflower for approximately 15 minutes.
2. In a large dish, blend the chives, salt, olive oil, parsley, garlic, pepper, and sour cream until combined.
3. Drain the hot water from the cauliflower and crush completely until the consistency is smooth.
4. Integrate the mixture to the cauliflower, totally blending.
5. Wait about 5 minutes before serving.

Pigs in a Blanket

Take a trip back your childhood with this fun low carb snack and even better if you get the kids to help!

Total Prep & Cooking Time: 40 minutes
Level: Beginner
Makes: 4 Helpings (3 Corn Dogs per serving)
Protein: 7 gram
Net Carbs: 3 grams
Fat: 26 grams
Sugar: 1 gram
Calories: 278

What you need:

1/8 cup heavy cream
Coconut oil spray
1/8 tsp salt
8 oz. almond flour
1/8 tsp garlic powder
3 tsp coconut flour
1/8 tsp onion powder
3/4 tsp baking powder, gluten-free

1/8 tsp pepper

3 tbs butter, salted and melted

1 large egg

2 beef hot dogs

1/8 cup water

Steps:

1. Set the oven to heat at 350° Fahrenheit. Use the coconut oil spray to lightly grease a mini cupcake tin.
2. In a big dish, whip the garlic powder, pepper, coconut flour, onion powder, and baking powder together removing any lumpiness.
3. Combine the eggs, almond flour, water, butter, heavy cream, and salt and totally incorporate the batter.
4. Let the mixture sit for approximately 3 minutes as it slightly thickens.
5. Evenly distribute into the prepped tin.
6. Slice each hot dog 6 times and place a piece into each of the poured dough.
7. Heat for approximately 20 minutes and remove to the counter.
8. Wait about 10 minutes before serving.

Baking Tip:
- Consider using beef or organic hot dogs for this recipe as conventional hot dogs usually have unwanted additives.

Radish Chips

If you are missing potato chips, these crispy radish chips might just be the ticket to your happy afternoon.

Total Prep & Cooking Time: 30 minutes
Level: Beginner
Makes: 4 Helpings
Protein: 1 gram
Net Carbs: 2 grams
Fat: 35 grams
Sugar: 2 grams
Calories: 350

What you need:

1/4 tbs onion powder
24 oz. extra virgin olive oil

1/4 tsp salt
48 oz. radishes, peeled & sliced
1/8 tsp pepper

Steps:

1. Peel and slice the radishes to your preferred thickness.
2. In a large skillet, warm the olive oil then reduce the temperature.
3. Fry the radishes for approximately 40 minutes if sliced thin, up to an hour if thicker. Sprinkle with the salt, onion powder and pepper and stir occasionally.
4. Remove to a paper towel covered platter and serve.

Baking Tip:
- If you want ultra-crispy chips, slice them thin and fry for approximately 50 minutes until the edges start to curl.

Spicy Deviled Eggs

This classic recipe that is a staple for any picnic or party has a kick that your taste buds will appreciate.

Total Prep & Cooking Time: 30 minutes
Level: Beginner
Makes: 4 Helpings
Protein: 6 grams
Net Carbs: 1.5 grams
Fat: 7 grams
Sugar: 1 gram
Calories: 94

What you need:

1/4 tsp cayenne pepper
2 large eggs, hardboiled
1/8 tsp cajun seasoning
4 thin slices of andouille sausage
1 tsp mustard
2 tsp mayonnaise, sugar-free
1/8 cup sauerkraut
1/4 tsp paprika

Steps:

1. Fill a small saucepan with 2 cups of the cold water to cover the eggs.
2. When the water begins to boil, set the timer for 7 minutes.
3. After the timer goes off, drain the water and cover the eggs with the remaining 2 cups of cold water.
4. Brown the sausage in a non-stick skillet until crispy. Remove to a platter covered in paper towels.
5. Peel and slice the eggs in halves long ways and transfer the yolks into a dish.
6. Combine the mayonnaise, cayenne pepper, Cajun seasoning, and mustard until smooth.
7. Place a slice of the sausage into the center of each egg and spoon the mixture on top of each.
8. Dust the top with paprika and serve.

Chapter 8: Dinner Recipes

Beef & Broccoli Stir fry

This stir fry meal is very easy to throw together even on a weeknight and tastes oh so yummy.

Total Prep & Cooking Time: 20 minutes plus 1 hour to marinate
Level: Beginner
Makes: 4 Helpings
Protein: 24 grams
Net Carbs: 6 grams
Fat: 26 grams
Sugar: 1 gram
Calories: 192

What you need:

For the main dish:

1/4 cup coconut oil
16 oz. flat iron steak
1 tsp toasted sesame oil
8 oz. broccoli, florets
1 tsp fish sauce

For the marinade:

1/8 cup tamari sauce, gluten-free
2 cloves garlic, chopped
1 tsp ginger, grated

Steps:

1. Slice the steak into quarter-inch pieces by cutting against the grain.
2. In a ziplock bag, combine the beef, tamari sauce, chopped garlic, and grated ginger. Refrigerate for an hour to marinate.
3. Boil the broccoli in a saucepan for approximately 2 minutes and drain as much water as possible.
4. Meanwhile, in a large skillet or wok, melt the coconut oil.
5. Remove the beef from the marinade and reserve the sauce for later.
6. When the pan is very hot, brown the beef for approximately 2 minutes and remove the meat to a plate.
7. Fry the broccoli in the wok for about 3 minutes and empty the marinade liquid into the pan. Allow to heat for 2 additional minutes.
8. Transfer the beef to the wok for approximately 90 seconds, stirring occasionally.

9. Drizzle the toasted sesame oil and fish sauce over the contents of the pan and serve.

Baking Tip:
- You may want to go straight to cooking without marinating the meat, but this will take away the amazing flavor that hour can give.

Variation Tips:
- Alternatively, you can use sirloin or flank steak in place of the flat iron steak.

Beef Kheema Meatloaf

This is an excellent twist on the conventional meatloaf recipe that is a brilliant way to use up that ground beef in your freezer.

Total Prep & Cooking Time: 25 minutes
Level: Beginner
Makes: 4 Helpings
Protein: 26 grams
Net Carbs: 5 grams
Fat: 13 grams
Sugar: 1 gram
Calories: 260

What you need:

16 oz. ground beef
1 tsp turmeric
2 large eggs
1 tbs onion powder

4 oz. cilantro, chopped

1 tsp salt

3 tsp ginger, minced

1 tsp cayenne pepper

3 tsp garlic, minced

1/2 tsp ground cinnamon

2 tsp garam masala

1/8 tsp ground cardamom

Air Fryer

Steps:

1. Set the temperature of the air fryer to heat at 360° Fahrenheit. Place an 8-inch heat safe round pan to the side.
2. In a food blender, combine all the listed components and pulse until thoroughly combined.
3. Distribute the meat evenly into the round pan and set the air fryer timer for 15 minutes.
4. After the time has passed, check with a meat thermometer to make sure it is at a uniform 160° Fahrenheit. If not, set for an additional 5 minutes.
5. Take out the pan and drain the meat.
6. Divide the meat into 4 equal servings and enjoy!

Baking Tip:
- If garam masala is not available, you can make your own! Simply add 1/2 tablespoon allspice and 1 1/2 tablespoon cumin seasonings.

Beef Stroganoff

This rendition of this definitive recipe has the typical creamy sauce and juicy beef without all the extra carbs.

Total Prep & Cooking Time: 30 minutes
Level: Intermediate/Expert
Makes: 4 Helpings
Protein: 28 grams
Net Carbs: 2.2 grams
Fat: 26 grams
Sugar: 0 grams
Calories: 410

What you need:

16 oz. beef steak, sirloin or tenderloin
3 tsp coconut oil
1 clove garlic, crushed
8 oz. heavy cream
1/2 tsp onion powder
4 oz. dry red wine

1/3 cup sour cream

8 oz. beef stock

1/4 tsp pepper, separated

2 tsp Dijon mustard

3 tsp chives, thinly sliced

1/2 tsp salt, separated

3 tsp parsley, chopped

Steps:

1. Slice the beef into sections approximately half an inch thick. Pat the sliced meat with a paper towel and set to the side.
2. Using a large non-stick skillet, heat the coconut oil, 1/4 teaspoon of salt, onion powder, garlic and 1/8 teaspoon of pepper.
3. Once the oil is warm, transfer the beef to the pan, but do not stir.
4. After about 2 minutes, flip the pieces of meat over to heat the alternate side.
5. Once both sides are seared, remove to a platter.
6. Lower the heat and empty the red wine in the pan. Swirl around the wine with a spoon for approximately 60 seconds while scraping the pan to deglaze.
7. Turn the heat back up to medium and let the wine reduce for an additional minute.
8. Move the meat back into the pan and mix with the reduced wine for about 90 seconds. Then turn the heat down to simmer.
9. Mix in the heavy cream thoroughly and allow the sauce to thicken over approximately 3 minutes.
10. Blend the sour cream, the remaining 1/8 teaspoon of pepper, Dijon mustard and the remaining 1/4 teaspoon of salt to the sauce until well combined.

11. Allow to simmer for 2 minutes and take away from the stove.
12. Garnish with chives and parsley and serve hot.

Baking Tip:
- Make sure that the slices of meat fit without going up the sides to ensure proper cooking. If the pan is too small, cook the meat in smaller batches.

Variation Tips:
- Alternatively, you can use beef tenderloin or sirloin in place of the beef steak.

- Instead of coconut oil, you may use a tablespoon of butter or ghee.

- If you enjoy mushrooms in your stroganoff, slice 8 ounces of your favorite mushrooms. After step 5, add an additional tablespoon of coconut oil or alternative and fry for approximately 2 minutes and remove to the plate with the meat. Add back into the pan in step 8.

Clam Chowder

This would be a wonderful dinner on a cold night and is surprisingly dairy free.

Total Prep & Cooking Time: 30 minutes
Level: Beginner
Makes: 4 Helpings
Protein: 2 grams
Net Carbs: 4 grams
Fat: 15 grams
Sugar: 2 grams
Calories: 164

What you need:

2 cups cauliflower florets
1 tsp onion powder
12 oz. steamer clams, shucked

1 1/3 tsp salt, separated
4 tbs butter, separated
1 1/3 cups water
13 oz. chicken broth
2 tsp rosemary
1/4 tsp pepper

Steps:

1. Using a deep saucepan, dissolve 2 tablespoons of butter.
2. Heat 1 1/2 cups of the cauliflower for about 2 minutes.
3. Empty the water, onion powder, 1 tablespoon of salt, chicken broth and remaining 2 tablespoons of butter into the saucepan and heat until bubbling.
4. Bring the heat down to medium, cover the pot with a lid and let it heat for about 10 minutes.
5. Remove the saucepan from the burner and transfer to a food blender. Pulse for approximately 60 seconds until a smooth consistency.
6. Distribute the mixture back to the saucepan and combine the remaining 1/2 cup of cauliflower, 1 teaspoon of rosemary and the clams.
7. Simmer for about 10 minutes and remove from the burner.
8. Season with pepper, the remaining teaspoon of salt and the remaining teaspoon of rosemary.

Baking Tip:
- Alternatively, you can substitute ghee for the butter.

Variation Tip:
- Garnish the chowder with a tablespoon of crushed bacon to add flavoring.

Chicken Kebab

When you sink your teeth into this flavorful shawarma, you will not be missing the bread that used to come with it.

Total Prep & Cooking Time: 45 minutes plus 2 hours to marinate
Level: Beginner
Makes: 4 Helpings
Protein: 35 grams
Net Carbs: 1 gram
Fat: 16 grams
Sugar: 0 grams
Calories: 274

What you need:

For the chicken:

21 oz. boneless chicken breast or thighs
2/3 tsp ground coriander

6 tsp olive oil

2/3 tsp ground cumin

1/3 tsp ground cayenne pepper

2/3 tsp ground cardamom

1/3 tsp garlic powder

2/3 tsp ground turmeric

1/3 tsp onion powder

2 tsp paprika powder

1 tsp salt

4 tsp lemon juice

1/8 tsp pepper

For the tahini sauce:

4 tsp olive oil

2 tbs water

1/3 tsp salt

4 tsp tahini paste

2 tsp lemon juice

1 clove garlic, minced

Steps:

1. With a rubber scraper, blend the coriander, olive oil, cumin, cayenne pepper, cardamom, garlic powder, turmeric, onion powder, paprika powder, salt, lemon juice and pepper in a big lidded tub.
2. Place the chicken inside and arrange, so they are covered completely by the liquid.
3. Marinate for at least 2 hours, if not overnight.
4. Preheat your grill to heat at 500° Fahrenheit.
5. Take away the chicken from the marinade and grill over the flames for approximately 4 minutes before flipping to the other side.
6. Grill until browned on both sides and use a meat thermometer to ensure it is a uniform 160° Fahrenheit.

7. Take away the chicken to a plate and cool for about 10 minutes.
8. In a small dish, blend the olive oil, water, salt, tahini paste, lemon, and minced garlic until a smooth consistency.
9. Slice the chicken and serve with the sauce and enjoy!

Baking Tips:

- If you do not own a grill, you can fry this meal on the stove. Once the chicken is marinated, dissolve a tablespoon of butter or coconut oil in a non-stick skillet. Fry the chicken on each side for approximately 4 minutes.

- Baking the chicken is another option. Adjust the temperature of the stove to 400° Fahrenheit and roast for approximately 20 minutes.

Variation Tip:

- If you like a kick to your chicken, you can add more cayenne pepper to your preferred taste.

Chicken Zucchini Meatballs

When you want an easy dinner, these meatballs will be quick to make after a hard day at work.

Total Prep & Cooking Time: 25 minutes
Level: Beginner
Makes: 4 Helpings
Protein: 26 grams
Net Carbs: 2.4 grams
Fat: 4 grams
Sugar: 1 gram
Calories: 161

What you need:

16 oz. chicken breasts, boneless
1/2 tsp celery seeds
2 cups zucchini, chopped
1 large egg
2 cloves garlic, peeled
1/2 tbs salt
3 tsp oregano
1/2 tsp pepper
2 tbs coconut oil

Steps:

1. Set the temperature of the stove to heat at 180° Fahrenheit. Layer a flat sheet with baking lining and set aside.
2. Use a food blender pulse all the components for approximately 3 minutes until totally incorporated.
3. Dissolve the coconut oil in a non-stick skillet.
4. Scoop out the meat and hand roll into one-inch meatballs.
5. Transfer to the hot oil and brown on each side for approximately 2 minutes.
6. Spoon the meatballs onto the prepped sheet and heat for about 10 minutes.
7. Serve warm and enjoy!

Chili Lime Drumsticks

Sink your teeth into this wonderful dinner that may just become your favorite flavorful meat on the Keto diet.

Total Prep & Cooking Time: 45 minutes plus 1 hour to marinate
Level: Beginner
Makes: 4 Helpings
Protein: 24 grams
Net Carbs: 1 gram
Fat: 15 grams
Sugar: 0 grams
Calories: 249

What you need:

1 tsp chili powder
4 chicken drumsticks
2 tsp lime juice
1 tsp garlic powder
3 tsp avocado oil
1/4 tsp salt

Steps:

1. In a big lidded tub, blend the chili powder, avocado oil, garlic powder, and lime juice until incorporated.
2. Place the meat into the liquid and arrange to cover completely.
3. Marinate for at least 60 minutes or overnight.
4. When you are ready to cook, adjust your grill to heat at 450° Fahrenheit.
5. Take away the chicken from the marinade and grill for about 35 minutes making sure to turn them over approximately every 5 minutes. Check the temperate with a meat thermometer until they reach 185° Fahrenheit.
6. Dust with salt and serve hot.

Egg Roll Bowl

Take out is not a thing of the past when you have this recipe to make in your own kitchen. And you do not even have to tip.

Total Prep& Cooking Time: 20 minutes
Level: Beginner
Makes: 4 Helpings
Protein: 29 grams
Net Carbs: 1 gram
Fat: 27 grams
Sugar: 0 grams
Calories: 376

What you need:

16 oz. ground sausage
1/2 tbs onion powder
4 cloves garlic, minced
1 tbs ginger, minced

4 cups cabbage, shredded
2 tsp tamari sauce, gluten-free
8 oz. mushrooms, sliced
1 tbs toasted sesame oil

Steps:

1. Brown the sausage in a non-stick skillet, crumbling the meat with a wooden spatula.
2. Combine the onion powder, ginger, tamari sauce, and garlic and stir for approximately 60 seconds.
3. Blend the mushrooms and cabbage into the skillet and blend with the spatula for about 3 additional minutes.
4. Remove from the burner and season with toasted sesame oil.
5. Serve immediately and enjoy!

Baking Tip:
- If you do not want to shred the cabbage yourself, you can use store bought shredded cabbage. Make sure there are not carrots included if you do not want to raise the carbs in the recipe.

Variation Tip:
- Substitute ground beef or turkey for variety.

- You can add a fried or boiled egg to the top of this salad if you need to raise your protein macros for the day.

Steak Plate & Veggies

This is a sheet pan recipe that makes dinner time a breeze. Enjoy this meat and veggie bomb tonight.

Total Prep & Cooking Time: 30 minutes
Level: Beginner
Makes: 4 Helpings
Protein: 28 grams
Net Carbs: 1.5 grams
Fat: 31 grams
Sugar: 0 grams
Calories: 384

What you need:

For Rosemary Caper Butter:

2 tsp rosemary, chopped
1/8 cup butter, softened
2 tsp capers, chopped
1 clove garlic, paste

For the main dish:

1 1/3 lbs. sirloin steak, approximately 1 inch thick
2 tbs olive oil, separated
1/2 tsp salt, separated
4 1/2 cups broccoli, florets
1/4 tsp pepper, separated
13 oz. asparagus spears

Steps:

1. Set the stove to the broil setting. Place a large flat sheet with a rim inside to heat.
2. In a glass dish, combine the pasted garlic, capers, butter and rosemary until smooth.
3. Transfer to a piece of plastic wrap, roll into a cylinder and refrigerate.
4. Use a paper towel to remove the excess moisture in the steaks and season with 1/8 teaspoon of pepper and 1/4 teaspoon of salt.
5. Place the broccoli and asparagus in a dish and cover fully with 1 tablespoon of olive oil, the remaining 1/8 teaspoon of pepper and the remaining 1/4 teaspoon of salt.
6. Remove the pan from the stove and brush with the remaining tablespoon of olive oil in the middle of the pan.
7. Put the meat on a pan with oil and garnish it with vegetables.
8. Heat for about 5 minutes and remove to flip the steaks to the other side.
9. Broil for an additional 5 minutes and remove to the counter.
10. Remove the butter from the fridge.
11. Butter the steaks and serve hot.

Walnut Chili

You will find that this chili is full of flavor with a couple of secret ingredients that make it stand out from the standard bowl you are used to.

Total Prep & Cooking Time: 45 minutes
Level: Beginner
Makes: 4 Helpings
Protein: 10 grams
Net Carbs: 5.6 grams
Fat: 13 grams
Sugar: 1 gram
Calories: 410

What you need:

1 tbs extra virgin olive oil
2 carrots, diced finely
1 tbs ground cinnamon
3 stalks celery, diced finely
1 tbs ground cumin
3 cloves garlic, minced
1 1/2 tsp paprika powder
2 large chipotle peppers, minced
1 1/2 cups walnuts, raw and minced
2 bell peppers, diced finely
1 1/2 oz. dark chocolate, unsweetened and chopped finely
30 oz. tomatoes, diced
1/4 tsp salt
2 1/2 cups tomato sauce
30 oz. black soybeans drained and rinsed
1/8 tsp pepper

Steps:

1. Using a large saucepan, liquefy the olive oil and combine the carrot and celery for approximately 4 minutes.
2. Blend the cumin, paprika, garlic, and cinnamon, stirring consistently for about 2 minutes.
3. Finally, combine the bell peppers, chipotle, tomato sauce, soy beans, walnuts, and tomatoes, stirring until fully incorporated.
4. Reduce the temperature to simmer for about 20 minutes or until the vegetables are fully cooked.
5. Melt the chocolate in the chili along with the pepper and salt.
6. Serve while still hot and enjoy!

Variation Tips:

- If you prefer spicy chili, add between 1 and 2 teaspoons of cayenne pepper.

- You can garnish your chili with avocado, cilantro leaves or sliced radishes to mix this recipe up.

Chapter 9: Unusual Delicious Meal Recipes

You have made it to the bonus chapter where there is a unique collection of recipes, as most are exotic and from overseas. Some have a few more steps, but they are still going to be easy enough for anyone to bring to their dinner table tonight. Enjoy experimenting with something new!

Blackberry Clafoutis Tarts

This rendition of the traditional dessert from France is very creamy and low carb to boot.

Total Prep & Cooking Time: 1 hour 30 minutes
Level: Beginner
Makes: 4 Tarts
Protein: 3 grams
Net Carbs: 2.4 grams

Fat: 15 grams
Sugar: 1 gram
Calories: 201

What you need:

For the crust:

1/4 cup coconut flour
2 tbs coconut oil, melted
2 tbs almond butter, smooth
1/4 tsp Swerve sweetener, confectioner
2 1/2 cups pecan pieces, raw
1/8 tsp salt

For the filling:

1 large egg
8 oz. blackberries
1/8 cup almond flour, blanched
2 oz. almond milk, unsweetened
3 tsp Stevia sweetener, granulated
1/8 tsp salt
3 oz. coconut milk, canned
1 tsp vanilla extract, sugar-free

Steps:

1. Set the stove to heat at 350° Fahrenheit. You will need to set aside four 4 3/4-inch tart pans.
2. To create the tart crusts, blend the coconut flour, Swerve, pecan pieces, salt, coconut oil, almond butter in a food blender for approximately 2 minutes until crumbly.
3. Scrape down the bowl with a rubber scraper and pulse for an additional 30 seconds.

4. Portion the batter in 4 equal sections and distribute to the tart pans. Press the crust evenly by starting with the sides with the middle being pressed last. Refrigerate to set for half an hour.
5. Remove the crusts from the fridge and place a quarter cup of blackberries in each tart pan.
6. Using the food blender, whip the Stevia, vanilla extract, egg, salt, coconut milk and almond milk for approximately half a minute.
7. Empty the contents evenly over the blackberries.
8. Heat the tarts for about half an hour and remove to the counter.
9. Wait approximately 10 minutes for serving warm. Enjoy!

Calamari Salad

This meal might look a little bit too unusual, but it will build your muscles after that powerful workout.

Total Prep & Cooking Time: 10 minutes
Level: Beginner
Makes: 4 Helpings
Protein: 18 grams
Net Carbs: 5 grams
Fat: 14 grams
Sugar: 0 grams
Calories: 214

What you need:

1/2 tsp lime juice
16 oz. calamari, sliced
1/4 tsp salt
2 tbs coconut oil
1/8 tsp pepper

8 oz. olives
1/2 tsp garlic powder
3 tsp coconut oil, separate
1/2 tsp lemon juice

Steps:

1. In a glass dish, blend the lemon and lime juice fully.
2. In a separate dish, whisk the 3 teaspoons of coconut oil, salt, garlic powder, and pepper until combined.
3. In a non-stick skillet, dissolve the 2 tablespoons of coconut oil with the olives. Heat the olives for about 90 seconds and remove to a serving plate.
4. Coat the calamari liberally in the seasonings.
5. Transfer the calamari to the hot oil and stir fry for approximately 2 minutes or until they become cloudy.
6. Remove to the serving plate with the olives.
7. Drizzle the juice dressing over the top of the plate and serve.

Carrot Pudding

Coming from the traditional Indian recipe books, this pudding is full of the healthy fats that your body needs to keep fueled.

Total Prep & Cooking Time: 45 minutes
Level: Beginner
Makes: 4 Helpings
Protein: 2 grams
Net Carbs: 1 gram
Fat: 18 grams
Sugar: 2 grams
Calories: 190

What you need:

3 cups carrots, grated
2 cups of coconut milk
1/2 tsp cardamom powder
2 1/2 tbs butter

6 tsp Erythritol sweetener, granulated

Steps:

1. Liquefy the butter and then simmer the carrots in a sauce pan until they become tender which will take approximately 8 minutes. Continuously stir the carrots, so they are fully cooked.
2. Empty the coconut milk into the saucepan, combining well.
3. Stir the carrots for an additional 15 minutes to ensure they do not stick.
4. Finally, blend the cardamom powder and Erythritol and heat until the milk has fully reduced.
5. Serve warm and enjoy.

Variation Tip:

- You can alternatively use ghee in this recipe in place of the butter.

- The traditional dish is usually topped with a few cashews.

Chicken Liver Pate

This is a traditional French dish that is loaded with healthy fats to help you liven up your Keto diet.

Total Prep & Cooking Time: 30 minutes plus 1 full day to marinate
Level: Beginner
Makes: 4 Helpings
Protein: 4 grams
Net Carbs: 2.3 grams
Fat: 11 grams
Sugar: 0 grams
Calories: 162

What you need:

8 oz. chicken liver
1/2 tbs apple cider vinegar
3 tsp coconut oil

1/2 tsp rosemary, stems removed

8 oz. green leek, chopped

1/4 tsp salt

2 tbs balsamic vinegar

1/2 tsp pepper

Steps:

1. Marinate the chicken liver in a combination of the apple cider vinegar and water in a glass baking dish for one full day.
2. Heat a cast iron skillet until the coconut oil is dissolved.
3. Drain the livers from the marinade and transfer to the pan with the leeks, salt, and rosemary, stirring to incorporate well.
4. Place a lid on the skillet and heat for about 10 minutes. The livers will be a little pink on the inside.
5. Remove from the burner and cool for approximately 5 minutes.
6. Empty the grease and livers into a food blender, scraping the skillet with a wooden spoon to remove all contents.
7. Pulse together with the pepper and balsamic vinegar until the consistency is silky.
8. Empty into a mason jar and serve immediately. Store in the refrigerator, and it will keep up to 4 days.

Eggplant Burger

This Chinese meal will add a decent amount of color to your dinner table and will build your muscles after your workout.

Total Prep & Cooking Time: 40 minutes
Level: Beginner
Makes: 4 Helpings
Protein: 26 grams
Net Carbs: 6 grams
Fat: 5 grams
Sugar: 0 grams
Calories: 205

What you need:

For the burgers:

1/2 lb. ground pork
2 Japanese eggplants
1/8 tsp pepper

2 tbs onion powder
1 tbs ginger, minced
2 tbs tamari sauce, gluten-free
1 tsp salt
Steaming Pot

For the sauce:

4 cloves of garlic, minced
1 tsp toasted sesame oil
4 tbs tamari sauce, gluten-free
1/2 tsp apple cider vinegar

Steps:

1. Chop the eggplant into sections about one inch thick. Make a slice to make them like an open bun, but not slicing all the way through.
2. Use a food blender to whip the ginger, ground pork, salt, onion powder, tamari sauce, and salt until combined fully.
3. Spoon the mixture evenly into the 4 sections of eggplant.
4. Transfer the burgers to a steamer and cook for approximately 20 minutes.
5. Meanwhile, in a glass serving dish, blend the garlic, toasted sesame oil, tamari sauce, and apple cider vinegar until smooth.
6. Remove the burgers from the steamer and place on a serving plate.
7. Serve immediately with the dipping sauce and enjoy!

Variation Tip:
- Instead of using tamari sauce, you can alternatively substitute 1/4 cup of coconut aminos.

Lobster Tails

You do not have to go to a fancy restaurant to have a flavorful meal at home.

Total Prep & Cooking Time: 25 minutes
Level: Beginner
Makes: 4 Helpings
Protein: 21 grams
Net Carbs: 5 grams
Fat: 14 grams
Sugar: 1 gram
Calories: 222

What you need:

4 lobster tails
2 tbs lemon juice
1 tsp Italian seasoning
5 cloves garlic, minced
4 tbs butter, melted

Steps:

1. Set the stove to heat at the temperature of 350° Fahrenheit. Using baking lining, cover a flat sheet and set aside.
2. In a glass dish, combine the melted butter, Italian seasoning, and garlic until integrated.
3. Remove the clear skin off the tail with sharp scissors.
4. Use a pastry brush to apply the butter mixture to the meat of the tails.
5. Move to the prepped sheet and heat in the stove for approximately 15 minutes. If you have larger tails, they will require an additional 5-10 minutes to fully cook.
6. Remove and enjoy hot.

Mediterranean Lamb Chops

Get a taste of the Mediterranean with this unique mix of spices that will really make your mouth water.

Total Prep & Cooking Time: 20 minutes
Level: Beginner
Makes: 4 Helpings (2 Chops per serving)
Protein: 29 grams
Net Carbs: 1 gram
Fat: 8 grams
Sugar: 1 gram
Calories: 164

What you need:

2 tsp lemon juice
1/4 tsp pepper
14 oz. lamb loin chops, trimmed and bone in

1/2 tsp extra virgin olive oil

2/3 tsp salt

1 1/2 cloves garlic, crushed

2 tsp Za'atar

Steps:

1. Heat the grill to the temperature of 350° Fahrenheit.
2. Prepare the lamb chops by brushing with garlic and oil.
3. Sprinkle the lemon juice over each side and dust with the salt, Za'atar, and pepper.
4. Grill on each side for approximately 4 minutes until your desired crispiness.

Baking Tip:

- Alternatively, you can broil in the stove for about 5 minutes on each side.

- If Za'atar seasoning is not available, you can easily make your own. You need the following ingredients:
  - 1/3 tbs oregano seasoning
  - 1/8 tsp sea salt
  - 1/3 tbs marjoram
  - 1/8 tbs roasted sesame seeds
  - 1/3 tbs thyme
  - 3 tbs sumac

Peanut Stew

Coming all the way from Africa, this is a popular dish that is filled with fats that will help keep you in ketosis.

Total Prep & Cooking Time: 25 minutes
Level: Beginner
Makes: 4 Helpings
Protein: 14 grams
Net Carbs: 6 grams
Fat: 26 grams
Sugar: 0 grams
Calories: 286

What you need:

For the stew:

16 oz. tofu, extra firm and cubed
1/4 tsp salt

3 tbs coconut oil
1/8 tsp pepper
3 tsp onion powder
1/2 tbs ginger, chopped finely

For the sauce:

4 tbs peanut butter
8 oz. vegetable broth, warmed
1/2 tsp turmeric
3 tsp sriracha
1 tsp paprika powder
4 oz. tomatoes, crushed
1/2 tsp cumin

Steps:

1. Heat the broth in a saucepan over medium heat. When boiling, remove from the burner.
2. Blend the sriracha, tomato sauce, cumin, turmeric, hot broth, peanut butter and paprika in the glass dish and integrate completely. It should thicken into a sauce. Set to the side.
3. Use a non-stick skillet to dissolve 2 tablespoons of coconut oil.
4. When the pan is hot, empty the cubes of tofu and brown on all sides taking approximately 4 minutes. Remove from the burner and transfer to a glass dish.
5. Combine the ginger, onion powder and the remaining tablespoon of coconut oil into the skillet and heat for 3 minutes.
6. Empty the browned tofu back into the skillet and continue to brown for an additional 2 minutes. Distribute into a serving bowl.

7. Dispense the sauce over the browned tofu and serve immediately.

Variation Tip:
- You can garnish this meal with a half a cup of dry roasted peanuts if you prefer more peanut taste.

Salmon Tartare

This would be the Keto diet´s version of raw fish sushi in this mini fat bomb that will have you smacking your lips.

Total Prep & Cooking Time: 25 minutes plus 2 hours to marinate (optional)
Level: Intermediate
Makes: 4 Helpings
Protein: 28 grams
Net Carbs: 1.8 grams
Fat: 40 grams
Sugar: 0 grams
Calories: 272

What you need:

16 oz. salmon fillet, skinless
5 oz. smoked salmon
1/4 tsp cayenne pepper

4 oz. mayonnaise, sugar-free

1/4 cup parsley, chopped

4 oz. extra virgin olive oil

2 tbs lime juice

1 tbs caper brine

2 tbs green olives, chopped

1/4 tsp pepper

2 tbs capers, chopped

1 tsp mustard, dijon

Steps:

1. Slice the smoked and fresh salmon into cubes about 1/4 inch wide and toss into a glass dish.
2. Blend the mayonnaise, cayenne pepper, chopped olives, pepper and mustard with the salmon until combined thoroughly.
3. Finally integrate the parsley, olive oil, lime juice, capers, and caper brine until incorporated fully.
4. Layer plastic wrap over the bowl and refrigerate for approximately 2 hours to marinate properly.
5. Remove the salmon from the fridge and section the fish into 4 servings.
6. Use a large circle cookie cutter to lightly push the salmon into a thick patty using a spoon.
7. Remove the cookie cutter and garnish with a splash of olive oil and serve.

Baking Tips:
- It is necessary to acquire fresh fish since this is a raw dish. If there is any skin on the salmon, it needs to be removed prior to cutting.

- Take care when cutting the fish into cubes. If you cut them too small, the tartare will be mushy.

- The marinating is not ultra-important to the dish, but it does help the ingredients to meld into each other properly.

Shrimp and Grits

This Southern tradition is a staple that can now be enjoyed on the Keto diet with this rendition of cauliflower grits.

Total Prep & Cooking Time: 40 minutes
Level: Beginner
Makes: 4 Helpings
Protein: 4 grams
Net Carbs: 5.3 grams
Fat: 11 grams
Sugar: 1 gram
Calories: 207

What you need:

For the topping:

16 oz. large shrimp, peeled and deveined
3 teaspoon butter
1/2 tsp thyme seasoning
2 cloves garlic, minced

1/4 tsp cayenne pepper

2 tsp paprika powder

1/4 tsp salt

For the grits:

3 cups cauliflower, florets

1/2 cup almond milk, unsweetened

3 tsp butter

1/4 tsp salt

3 tsp nutritional yeast

1 cup of water

Steps:

1. Heat the cauliflower in a large pot with the water. Once the water begins to boil, cover with a lid and set a timer for 20 minutes.
2. Check the cauliflower with a fork to ensure it is cooked thoroughly.
3. Drain the water from the pot and transfer the cauliflower to a food blender.
4. Combine the nutritional yeast, salt, butter and almond to the blender and pulse for approximately 2 minutes until the consistency is very smooth.
5. Combine paprika powder, cayenne pepper, garlic and thyme, and in a small dish and whisk to integrate.
6. Combine the mixed spices in a skillet along with the hot coconut oil.
7. Detach the tails and eliminate the moisture from the shrimp by dabbing with a paper towel.
8. Brown the shrimp for approximately 9 minutes while occasionally stirring.
9. Meanwhile, distribute the grits into a serving bowl and

once the shrimp are pink, empty the whole contents of the pan on top of the grits.

Baking Tip:

- You may also use frozen shrimp for this recipe. Ensure they have completely thawed ahead of time and decrease the frying time by 3 minutes.

Variation Tip:

- Add a garnish of lemon juice, chives or a splash of hot sauce.

- Ghee will work as a substitute for the butter in this meal.

Index for the Recipes

Spicy Deviled Eggs

Chapter 8: Dinner Recipes

Beef & Broccoli Stir fry
Beef Kheema Meatloaf
Beef Stroganoff
Clam Chowder
Chicken Kebab
Chicken Zucchini Meatballs
Chili Lime Drumsticks
Egg Roll Bowl
Steak Plate & Veggies
Walnut Chili

Chapter 9: Unusual Meal Recipes

Blackberry Clafoutis Tarts
Calamari Salad
Carrot Pudding
Chicken Liver Pate
Eggplant Burger
Lobster Tails
Mediterranean Lamb Chops
Peanut Stew
Salmon Tartare
Shrimp & Grits

Made in the USA
Columbia, SC
19 June 2019